TRAINING DAY

TRAINING DAY

400+ *ORIGINAL* WORKOUTS TO INCORPORATE IN YOUR TRAINING

CHIPPERS • INTERVALS • RUNNING • COUPLETS • TRIPLETS
AMRAPS • BODYWEIGHT • GYMNASTICS • PARTNER • & MORE!

DAMECT DOMINGUEZ

Copyright © 2017 Damect Dominguez

All rights reserved. No part of this book may be reproduced or transmitted in any form or by any means, without permission in writing from the publisher.

Published in the United States of America

First Edition, December 2017

Book/Cover Design by Damect Dominguez

To my grandmother, Mateta
& my mother, Mayita.

CONTENTS

INTRODUCTION:
PROGRAMMING YOUR WORKOUTS — 10
  STRUCTURING A WEEK — 10
  SAMPLE WEEK — 12
  STRUCTURING A YEAR — 13
  IMPORTANT WOD NOTES — 15

CHAPTER ONE:
COUPLETS — 19

CHAPTER TWO:
TRIPLETS — 29

CHAPTER THREE:
AMRAPS — 42

CHAPTER FOUR:
FOR TIME — 54

CHAPTER FIVE:
INTERVALS — 71

CHAPTER SIX:
GYMNASTICS — 89

CHAPTER SEVEN:
BODYWEIGHT — 97

CHAPTER EIGHT:
PARTNER — 106

CHAPTER NINE:
CHIPPERS — 128

CHAPTER TEN (A):
RUNNING — 139

CHAPTER TEN (B)
LONG INTERVAL RUNNING — 145

INTRODUCTION
PROGRAMMING YOUR WORKOUTS

In total, you'll find over 400 WODs (Workout of the Day) in this book. These workouts can be used 'grab-and-go' style, where on any given day, you randomly, or based on the type of workout you feel like doing that day, select a WOD and *go*. The WODs in this book can also be used in a more methodical and structured way, creating a program that consistently targets different energy systems and skill sets. Your body, when treated correctly and provided with stimuli in the correct way, adapts to the stressors provided to it in training. Want to get stronger? Stress (train) your body with the appropriate loads at the right times (intensity, volume, and frequency).

STRUCTURING A WEEK
Frequency
The first aspect to determine is your training frequency, or how often you'll be training. I recommend you stick to a 3/1/2/1 approach (3 days on, 1 day off followed by 2 days on, 1 day off). Not only does this structure work better with most people's schedules, it's been proven effective in a variety of functional fitness, running, bodybuilding, and other fitness programs. Of course, depending on your unique needs, you can structure your week on a 3 days on, 1 day off or a 5 days on, 2 days off approach.

Daily Volume
When structuring a week, daily volume is of particular importance. If we give total volume for the week a value of 24, I recommend structuring daily volume as such:

Monday: 4
Tuesday: 6
Wednesday: 5
Thursday: 0 (rest)

Friday: 4
Saturday: 5
Sunday: 0 (rest)

In this distribution of volume, Tuesday is the highest volume day followed by Wednesday and Saturday. Monday and Friday are the lowest volume days. Begin with these daily volume recommendations and as you become better acquainted with your abilities, adjust as needed.

Selecting Workouts
The goal of any functional fitness program is to create a well-rounded athlete. As such, you have to pay particular attention to modalities trained (gymnastics, weightlifting, and monostructural exercises like running, rowing and biking), time domains (a five-minute WOD versus a 20-minute WOD, for example), sets and reps, and intensity.

Weekly Guidelines for Selecting Workouts
- 3-4 WODs under 14 minutes; if possible, 1 of those under 6 minutes.
- 1 WOD longer than 14 minutes
- 3 WODs with gymnastics and weightlifting components, respectively
- At least 1 WOD from the Gymnastics chapter
- 1-2 barbell intensive WOD
- At least 1 WOD with running, rowing, or biking as the main component
- 1-2 Interval WODs
- 1-2 heavy WODs; if possible, on either Monday or Friday
- At least 1 WOD from the Bodyweight chapter
- Every 2 weeks, 1 WOD longer than 30 minutes

SAMPLE WEEK

Monday
TRIPLET WOD 43
21 Calorie Bike
15 Squat Cleans
9 Shoulder-to-Overhead
Bar Weight: 185/130

Tuesday
GYMNASTICS WOD 7
5 Rounds
45 Double-unders
15 Handstand Push-ups

AMRAP WOD 3
8 Minute AMRAP
4 Deadlifts (225/155)
10 Russian Kettlebell Swings (70/53)
5 Box Jumps (30/24)

Wednesday
INTERVAL WOD 34
24 Minute EMOM
M1: 10 Dumbbell Squat Snatches (50/35)
M2: 15 GHD Sit-ups
M3: 20 Bar Thrusters (45/35)
M4: 12/10 Calorie Bike

Thursday
Rest Day

Friday
FOR TIME WOD 10
5 Rounds
9 Power Cleans (135/95)
12 Toes-to-Bar

Saturday
BODYWEIGHT WOD 7
5 Rounds
50 Double-unders
10 Ring Dips
10 Ring Push-ups

RUNNING WOD 1
For Time
1,000 Meter Row
400 Meter Run
500 Meter Row
400 Meter Run

Sunday
Rest Day

STRUCTURING A YEAR

Structuring a 52-week training plan can be a daunting process. Fortunately, by dividing your year into different phases and periodizing your training, things become much easier. This training method helps you move progressively from one phase to the next, resulting in a peak fitness stage at the end. Periodizing your training also provides variety and sufficient periods of rest, both necessary components in avoiding plateaus and overtraining. This 52-week training plan will be broken up into two training cycles; each training cycle will have 3-4 phases (depending on the athlete) and will last approximately 26 weeks.

The Four Phases

FOUNDATION (3-6 WEEKS)

This period is encouraged for new athletes. During this phase, athletes should start getting familiar with all the movements in this book and prepping their mind and body for regular training. Athletes can begin to incorporate workouts they feel comfortable with; the Bodyweight chapter is a great place to start.

BASE BUILDING (12-16 WEEKS)

This period is focused on building a strong aerobic, strength, and gymnastics skill base. Just as you needed the foundation phase (at some point in your training) to be able to advance your training, you'll need this phase to move more efficiently later on in the year. Depending on your individual weaknesses, you may want to have a slight focus toward either building an aerobic or strength base or improving your gymnastics. Incorporating a supplemental strength program during this phase is highly recommended. Be sure that whatever strength program you choose, it works well when incorporated into a functional fitness program like this. During this period, your volume should build for three weeks and back off for one in order to allow your body to properly recover. This is an important phase for all athletes, but beginner athletes should consider spending more time in this phase as this is where you'll gain enough fitness to handle higher levels of intensity in the next phase.

Weekly Guidelines for Selecting Workout in the Base Phase
- 2-3 WODs under 12 minutes
- 2-3 WODs longer than 15 minutes (alternate between 2 and 3 WODs on a weekly basis)
- 3 WODs with gymnastics and weightlifting components, respectively
- 2 WODs with a heavy focus on running, biking, or rowing
- At least 2-3 WODs from the Gymnastics chapter
- 1 barbell intensive WOD
- 1-2 Interval WODs
- 1 heavy WOD
- At least 2 WODs from the Bodyweight chapter

INTENSITY (6-8 WEEKS)

The goal of the Intensity phase is to maximize your fitness by gradually increasing intensity while reducing total training volume. Trust that the previous phases have improved the quality of your movements, your aerobic base, and your mental capacity to push it in a WOD. Just like you did in the Base Building phase, decrease volume every fourth week to allow for proper recovery.

Weekly Guidelines for Selecting Workout in the Intensity Phase
- 2-3 WODs under 14 minutes
- 2-3 WODs under 6 minutes
- 1 WOD over 20 minutes
- 3-4 WODs with gymnastics and weightlifting components, respectively
- 2-3 barbell intensive WODs.
- 1 heavy WOD

RECOVERY (2-4 WEEKS)
After finishing approximately 22 weeks of intense training, it's time to let your body recover. During this time, you'll continue to train, but reduce the volume and intensity significantly. Don't worry about selecting workouts based on any particular plan. Instead, choose workouts based on how you feel that specific day. Remember, this is the time to rest your body *and* your mind—stay active but focused on recovery.

IMPORTANT WOD NOTES
1. Reading a Typical WOD

Couplet WOD 4
3 Rounds
5 Power Cleans (185/130)
7 Box Jumps (30/24)

What it means: To complete Couplet WOD 4, athletes will work through 3 rounds of 5 power cleans at 185lbs for the men and 130lbs for the women and 7 box jumps at 30 inches for the men and 24 inches for the women. The first number in parenthesis will always denote the men's weight/height while the second number will denote the women's weight/height.

Couplet WOD 13
21-15-9
Calorie Row
Power Snatches (95/65)

What it means: To complete Couplet WOD 13, athletes will work through 3 rounds of calorie row and power snatches. Round 1 will consist of 21 reps of both movements, round 2 will consist of 15 reps of both movements, and the final round will consist of 9 reps of both movements. The workout will look as follows:

21 Calorie Row
21 Power Snatches

15 Calorie Row
15 Power Snatches
9 Calorie Row
9 Power Snatches

2. Scaling a Workout

The beauty of the workouts in this book is that they are scalable to athletes of all levels. If you're able to do the workouts in this book as prescribed (without needing to adjust any of the weights, reps, or movements), perfect—you're all set to go. A word of caution though—many athletes get caught up in doing WODs Rx (as prescribed or as they are written) to realize a sense of achievement or to satisfy the ego. However, doing a workout as prescribed is only to be celebrated if *both* the intensity of the workout is preserved and movement quality is maintained. If you haven't reached Rx status, don't worry! Despite individual athlete limitations such as experience, injury, or fitness level, everyone should be able to get the same intended stimuli from a workout if scaled properly. Like most concepts in life, the more experience you get scaling workouts, the better you'll be at it.

The options for scaling workouts are plentiful. Remember, any part of the workout can be scaled: reps, weights, and movements. More often it's the latter two that athletes adjust—weights and movements. Let's take a look at a couple of examples:

Couplet WOD 22
27-21-15-9
Overhead Squats (95/65)
Toes-to- Bar

Couplet WOD 22 is intended to be fairly light; this will *usually* be the case when the rep scheme is high. Let's say the weight (95/65) is heavy enough that you'll have to do four to five reps at a time to complete the opening set of 27 overhead squats—in which case you'll definitely be sacrificing the intended intensity of the workout.

So, it makes sense to drop the weight of the overhead squats to 65/45, for example. If you can move that weight at a higher intensity (for example, breaking the opening set of 27 overhead squats in no more than two or three sets) without sacrificing form, then you've probably scaled properly. Scaling is an art, not a science! As for the toes-to-bar, if you don't have them yet, or if you aren't proficient enough at them to do them in a workout, you can scale them by replacing them with butterfly sit-ups, knees-to-elbow, or GHD sit-ups, to name a few.

AMRAP WOD 13
9 Minute AMRAP
3 Hang Power Snatches (165/115)
6 Strict Handstand Push-ups

Whereas Couplet WOD 22 was intended to be fairly light, this one is meant to be moderately heavy. Personally, I would recommend scaling the weight on the hang power snatches to the heaviest possible weight you can do three times, without breaking, while maintaining good form. You may want to go a little heavier even if you have to resort to singles. Both scaling options would be acceptable as long as you move with relative intensity through the singles. If you have to rest a minute or more between each rep, you've probably gone too heavy. If you need to replace the strict handstand push-ups, you can do so with push-ups, kipping handstand push-ups, handstand holds, or strict presses, to name a few options.

CHAPTER 1
COUPLETS

A couplet is a workout that pairs two functional movements—push-ups and pull-ups, for example. The simplicity of a couplet however, is no indication of its effectiveness or how difficult or easy it is to complete. As a matter of fact, couplets (and triplets, for that matter) are so effective that they should actually make up the majority of your workouts. As for the difficulty of these workouts, in the CrossFit community, couplets are often regarded as some of the most brutal workouts.

When programmed correctly, the two movements in a couplet should complement each other in any number of ways. One common way is to build on the concept of push and pull. A couplet workout creates a sense of rest by targeting one area or one muscle group for the first movement, then allowing it to rest by utilizing a different group of muscles for the second movement. A workout with push-ups and pull-ups is a perfect example of this. The push-ups target your pushing muscles, primarily your chest and triceps, while the pull-ups target your pulling muscles, primarily your back and biceps.

Another concept used throughout this chapter to program couplets includes pairing a traditional weightlifting movement like the snatch with a gymnastics movement like pull-ups or toes-to-bar or with a monostructural metabolic conditioning movement like rowing or running. While not all the workouts in this chapter subscribe to the concepts mentioned here, they all stay true to the intent of a couplet workout—forcing you to go back to a movement round after round, under increasing fatigue, after completing just one other movement. While all couplets can have either a task or time priority, all the workouts in this chapter have a task priority. The *For Time* chapter will include couplets with a time priority.

COUPLET WOD 1
4 Rounds
20 Wall Balls (20/14)
10 Hang Power Snatches (95/65)

COUPLET WOD 2
2 Rounds
30 Power Cleans (135/95)
50 Wall Balls

COUPLET WOD 3
4 Rounds
12 Deadlifts (185/130)
10 Pull-ups

COUPLET WOD 4
3 Rounds
5 Power Cleans (185/130)
7 Box Jumps (30/24)

COUPLET WOD 5
4 Rounds
15 Overhead Squats (95/65)
15/12 Calorie Bike

COUPLET WOD 6
4 Rounds
3 Complexes of 1 Snatch + 1 Hang Snatch (165/115)
30 Double-unders
You may not drop the bar once you begin the complex.

COUPLET WOD 7
3 Rounds
20 Kettlebell Swings (53/35)
10 Box Jumps (24/20)

COUPLET WOD 8
40-30-20
Thrusters (45/35)
Calorie row

COUPLET WOD 9
6 Rounds
15/12 Calorie Bike
40 Double-unders

FOR TIME WOD 10
5 Rounds
9 Power Cleans (135/95)
12 Toes-to-Bar

COUPLET WOD 11
3 Rounds
10 Deadlifts (225/155)
15 Wall Balls (30/20)

COUPLET WOD 12
3 Rounds
12 Power Cleans (135/95)
15 Burpee Box Jumps (24/20)

COUPLET WOD 13
21-15-9
Calorie Row
Power Snatches (95/65)

COUPLET WOD 14
3 Rounds
25/20 Calorie Bike
30 Wall Balls (24/20)

COUPLET WOD 15
21-15-9
Deadlifts (185/130)
Chest-to-Bar Pull-ups

COUPLET WOD 16
4 Rounds
15/12 Calorie Bike
20 Shoulder-to-Overhead (95/65)

COUPLET WOD 17
3 Rounds
15 Power Cleans (135/95)
30 Double-unders

COUPLET WOD 18
4 Rounds
2 Complexes of 2 Squat Cleans + 1 Jerk* (235/165)
6 Over-the- Bar Burpees
*You may not drop the bar once you begin the complex.

COUPLET WOD 19
3 15' Legless Rope Climbs
10 Squat Cleans

2 15' Legless Rope Climbs
8 Squat Cleans

1 15' Legless Rope Climb
6 Squat Cleans
Bar Weight: 185/130

COUPLET WOD 20
4 Rounds
3 Squat Snatches (185/130)
6 Over-the-Bar Burpees

COUPLET WOD 21
40 Thrusters
5 Bar Muscle-Ups

30 Thrusters
8 Bar Muscle-Ups

20 Thrusters
11 Bar Muscle-Ups

10 Thrusters
13 Bar Muscle-Ups
Bar Weight: 45/35

COUPLET WOD 22
27-21-15-9
Overhead Squats (95/65)
Toes-to- Bar

COUPLET WOD 23
15-12-9
Push Presses (135/95)
Over-the-Bar Burpees

COUPLET WOD 24
10 Rounds
5 Thrusters (95/65)
5 Box Jumps (24/20)

COUPLET WOD 25
21-15-9
Deadlifts (185/130)
Bar Facing Over-the-Bar Burpees

COUPLET WOD 26
5 Rounds
9 Thrusters (95/65)
4 Ring Muscle-Ups

COUPLET WOD 27
3 Rounds
250 Meter Row
10 Kettlebell Swings (70/53)

COUPLET WOD 28
4 Rounds
10 Alternating Dumbbell Squat Snatches (50/35)*
10 Strict Pull-Ups
*5 dumbbell snatches on each arm per round.

COUPLET WOD 29
10 Rounds
4 Power Snatches (115/80)
4 Box Jumps (24/20)

COUPLET WOD 30
3 Rounds
10 Power Cleans (185/130)
20 Wall Balls (20/14)

COUPLET WOD 31
15 Thrusters
40 Double-unders

10 Thrusters
30 Double-unders

5 Thrusters
20 Double-unders
Bar Weight: 135/95

COUPLET WOD 32
50 Wall Balls
25 Kettlebell Swings

35 Wall Balls
25 Kettlebell Swings

20 Wall Balls
25 Kettlebell Swings
Wall Balls: 20/14
Kettlebell Swings: 70/53

COUPLET WOD 33
9-6-3
Deadlifts (315/220)
Bar Muscle-ups

COUPLET WOD 34
40/32 Calorie Bike
21 Thrusters

30/24 Calorie Bike
15 Thrusters

20/16 Calorie Bike
9 Thrusters

10/8 Calorie Bike
3 Thrusters
Bar Weight: 95/65

COUPLET WOD 35
6 Rounds
8 Shoulder-to-Overhead (115/80)
40 Double-unders

COUPLET WOD 36
3 Rounds
15/12 Calorie Bike
10 Clean + Jerks (135/95)

COUPLET WOD 37
5 Rounds
10 Deadlifts (225/155)
4 15' Rope Climbs

COUPLET WOD 38
30 Hang Snatches (115/80)
40 Chest-to-Bar Pull-ups

COUPLET WOD 39
5 Rounds
5 Squat Snatches (135/95)
5 Ring Muscle-ups

COUPLET WOD 40
21 Power Cleans
15 Handstand Push-ups

15 Power Cleans
12 Handstand Push-ups

9 Power Cleans
9 Handstand Push-ups

3 Power Cleans
6 Handstand Push-ups
Bar Weight: 135/95

COUPLET WOD 41
15-9-6-3
Power Snatches (95/65)
Over-the-Bar Burpees

COUPLET WOD 42
4 Rounds
40 Air Squats
20 Kettlebell Swings (70/53)

COUPLET WOD 43
50 Thrusters
30/24 Calorie Row

40 Thrusters
20/16 Calorie Row

30 Thrusters
20/14 Calorie Row
Bar Weight: 45/35

COUPLET WOD 44
21-15-9
Thrusters (95/65)
Push-ups

COUPLET WOD 45
4 Rounds
12 Overhead Squats (115/80)
4 15' Rope Climbs

COUPLET WOD 46
4 Rounds
5 Deadlifts (335/235)
10 Handstand Push-ups

CHAPTER 2
TRIPLETS

A triplet is similar in design to a couplet, but pairs three functional movements instead of two. The inclusion of a third movement allows for more variety, movement patterns and a broader test of fitness. Does this make a triplet better than a couplet? Not necessarily. However, triplets do add an important layer to any functional fitness program. With the inclusion of triplets, we can add workouts that incorporate all three modalities (gymnastics and bodyweight, monostructural metabolic conditioning, and weightlifting), for example. As I stated in the previous chapter, triplets (along with couplets) should make up the majority of your workouts.

Triplet WOD 25
21-15-9
Calorie Row *(monostructural metabolic conditioning)*
Power Cleans (135/95) *(weightlifting)*
Pull-ups *(gymnastics)*

We can also program workouts to have a slight or complete bias toward one of the modalities. Triplet WOD 1, for example, has a weightlifting bias while Triplet WOD 46 has a slight gymnastics bias.

Triplet WOD 1	**Triplet WOD 47**
Weightlifting Bias	*Gymnastics Bias*
4 Rounds	4 Rounds
10 Power Cleans	8 Chest-to-Bar Pull-ups
8 Front Squats	10 Overhead Squats (95/65)
10 Toes-to-Bar	8 Toes-to-Bar
Bar Weight: 135/95	

As was the case with the couplets, while all triplets can have either a task or time priority, all the workouts in this chapter have a task priority. The *For Time* chapter will include triplets with a time priority.

TRIPLET WOD 1
4 Rounds
10 Power Cleans
8 Front Squats
10 Toes-to-Bar
Bar Weight: 135/95

TRIPLET WOD 2
4 Rounds
30 Double-unders
8 Deadlifts (225/155)
10 Pull-ups

TRIPLET WOD 3
5 Rounds
20 Wall Balls (20/14)
10 Box Jumps (24/20)
10 Calorie Bike

TRIPLET WOD 4
21-15-9
Deadlifts (225/155)
Over-the-Bar Burpees
Handstand Push-ups

TRIPLET WOD 5
4 Rounds
8 Thrusters (135/95)
15 Calorie Row
5 Bar Muscle-ups

TRIPLET WOD 6
15 Power Snatches
20 Overhead Squats
60 Double-unders

12 Power Snatches
15 Overhead Squats
50 Double-unders

9 Power Snatches
10 Overhead Squats
40 Double-unders

6 Power Snatches
5 Overhead Squats
30 Double-unders
Bar Weight: 115/80

TRIPLET WOD 7
21-15-9
Calorie Row
Front Squats
Shoulder-to-Overhead
Bar Weight: 135/95

TRIPLET WOD 8
4 Rounds
10 Kettlebell Thrusters (53/35)*
20 Russian Kettlebell Swings (40/25)
30 Double-unders
Use 2 kettlebells, one in each hand.

TRIPLET WOD 9
3 Rounds
10 Squat Cleans (135/95)
8 Over-the-Bar Burpees
10 Kettlebell Swings (70/53)

TRIPLET WOD 10
4 Rounds
10 Chest-to-Bar Pull-ups
15 Power Snatches (75/55)
40 Double-unders

TRIPLET WOD 11
40 Power Cleans
40 Shoulder-to-Overhead
40 Front Squats
Bar Weight: 135/95

TRIPLET WOD 12
15 Overhead Squats
8 Ring Muscle-ups
15 Over-the-Bar Burpees

20 Overhead Squats
6 Ring Muscle-ups
12 Over-the-Bar Burpees

25 Overhead Squats
4 Ring Muscle-ups
9 Over-the-Bar Burpees
Bar Weight: 95/65

TRIPLET WOD 13
2 Rounds
20 Kettlebell Swings (70/53)
30 Wall Balls (20/14)
10 Box Jumps (24/20)

TRIPLET WOD 14
21-15-9
Deadlifts (225/155)
Box Jumps (24/20)
Calorie Row

TRIPLET WOD 15
3 Rounds
5 Snatches (135/95)
8 Chest-to-Bar Pull-ups
2 15' Rope Climbs

TRIPLET WOD 16
5 Rounds
10 Calorie Bike
7 Power Cleans (135/95)
4 Bar Muscle-ups

TRIPLET WOD 17
21-15-9
Thrusters (95/65)
Box Jumps (24/20)
Calorie Bike

TRIPLET WOD 18
3 Rounds
10 Clean + Jerks (135/95)
20 Med Ball GHD Sit-Ups (14/10)
25-Yard Slamball Bear Hug Carry (100/70)

TRIPLET WOD 19
25-20-15-10
Pull-Ups
Snatches (75/55)
Calorie Row

TRIPLET WOD 20
21-15-9
Shoulder-to-Overhead (95/65)
Double-unders
Calorie Bike

TRIPLET WOD 21
3 Rounds
12 Handstand Push-ups
16 Deadlifts (225/155)
20 Double-unders

TRIPLET WOD 22
4 Rounds
40 Double-unders
15 Power Snatches (95/65)
10 Chest-to-Bar Pull-ups

TRIPLET WOD 23
27-21-15-9
Dumbbell Squat Cleans (50/35)*
Chest-to-Bar Pull-ups
Burpees
One dumbbell in each hand.

TRIPLET WOD 24
4 Rounds
8 Deadlifts (275/190)
10 Chest-to-Bar Pull-ups
25 Double-unders

TRIPLET WOD 25
21-15-9
Calorie Row
Power Cleans (135/95)
Pull-ups

TRIPLET WOD 26
25-20-15
Snatches (95/65)
Calorie Row
Russian Kettlebell Swings (70/53)

TRIPLET WOD 27
21-15-9
Back Squats (165/115)
Box Jumps (24/20)
Calorie Row

TRIPLET WOD 28
5 Rounds
10 Squat Snatches
10 Overhead Squats
10 Box Jumps (24/20)
Bar Weight: 135/95

TRIPLET WOD 29
3 Rounds
8 Deadlifts (275/190)
30 Double-unders
8 Box Jumps (24/20)

TRIPLET WOD 30
3 Rounds
10 Power Snatches (95/65)
10 Over-the-Bar Burpees
10 Box Jumps (24/20)

TRIPLET WOD 31
3 Rounds
12 Power Cleans
12 Push Presses
12 Thrusters
Bar Weight: 95/65

TRIPLET WOD 32
4 Rounds
20-Yard Back Rack Lunges (135/95)
10 Over-the-Bar Burpees
30 Double-unders

TRIPLET WOD 33
40-30-20
Thrusters (75/55)
Calorie Row
Double-unders

TRIPLET WOD 34
4 Rounds
5 Squat Cleans (255/180)
10 Handstand Push-ups
5 Bar Muscle-ups

TRIPLET WOD 35
4 Rounds
12 Power Snatches (115/80)
14 Wall Balls (30/20)
16 Kettlebell Swings (70/53)

TRIPLET WOD 36
4 Rounds
20 Goblet Squats (70/53)
15 Push Press (115/80)
10 Box Jumps (30/24)

TRIPLET WOD 37
21-15-9
Calorie Bike
Back Squats (185/130)
Toes-to-Bar

TRIPLET WOD 38
4 Rounds
15 Hang Snatches (115/80)
10 Box Jumps (24/20)
5 Muscle-ups

TRIPLET WOD 39
30 Dumbbell Thrusters
20 Box Jumps
50 Double-unders

20 Dumbbell Thrusters
15 Box Jumps
50 Double-unders

10 Dumbbell Thrusters
10 Box Jumps
50 Double-unders
Dumbbells: 30/20
Box Jump Height: 24/20
Use two dumbbells for the thrusters.

TRIPLET WOD 40
5 Rounds
6 Thrusters (115/80)
8 Over-the-Bar Burpees
10 Calorie Bike

TRIPLET WOD 41
3 Rounds
40 Air Squats
30 Snatches (75/55)
20 Burpee Box Jump Overs (24/20)

TRIPLET WOD 42
5 Rounds
10 Toes-to-Bar
12 Dumbbell Snatches, Alternating Hands (50/35)*
14 Calorie Row

TRIPLET WOD 43
3 Rounds
10 Power Cleans (155/110)
15 Pull-ups
20 Russian Kettlebell Swings (70/53)

TRIPLET WOD 44
3 Rounds
12 Shoulder-to-Overhead
10 Ring Dips
8 Hang Power Cleans
Bar Weight: 135/95

TRIPLET WOD 45
4 Rounds
3 Hang Snatches
6 Overhead Squats
9 Toes-to-Bar
Bar Weight: 115/80

TRIPLET WOD 46
8 Rounds
5 Thrusters (95/65)
5 Box Jumps (24/20)
10 Russian Kettlebell Swings (70/53)

TRIPLET WOD 47
4 Rounds
8 Chest-to-Bar Pull-ups
10 Overhead Squats (95/65)
8 Toes-to-Bar

TRIPLET WOD 48
20 Overhead Squats (95/65)
10 Strict Pull-ups
10 Toes-to-Bar

TRIPLET WOD 49
5 Rounds
6 Thrusters (115/80)
8 Over-the-Bar Burpees
10 Calorie Bike

TRIPLET WOD 50
3 Rounds
40 Air Squats
30 Snatches (75/55)
20 Burpee Box Jump Overs

TRIPLET WOD 51
21-15-9
Dumbbell Squat Cleans (50/35)*
Chest-to-Bar Pull-ups
Burpees
*Use two dumbbells.

TRIPLET WOD 52
21 Calorie Bike
15 Squat Cleans
9 Shoulder-to-Overhead
Bar Weight: 185/130

TRIPLET WOD 53
40-30-20-10
Overhead Squats (95/65)
Calorie Bike
Handstand Push-ups

TRIPLET WOD 54
21-15-9
Kettlebell Squat Snatch, Alternating Hands (53/35)
Burpees
Bike Calories

CHAPTER 3
AMRAPS

AMRAPs are time limit workouts where the goal is to complete As Many Reps (or Rounds) As Possible. This type of workout possesses a unique set of benefits that make them a necessary component in any well-rounded workout program.

Let's take a closer look. An AMRAP, for example, may require an athlete to complete as many reps as possible of: 12 burpees, 10 butterfly sit-ups, and 8 air squats in 12 minutes. Notice that there's no minimum or maximum work required; an athlete can complete 32 reps (1 full round) or 100 reps (3.125 rounds). The total number of reps completed will be unique to each athlete. The common denominator is that all athletes should push themselves as hard as possible for the duration of the workout.

The makeup of an AMRAP caters very well to novice athletes. It's arguably the simplest workout concept you'll find in this book—work as hard as possible for X number of minutes. For more experienced athletes, AMRAPs should be consistently incorporated in training as well. As a matter of fact, they're one of the most popular forms of training in CrossFit, and make up the majority of workouts in the CrossFit Open (CrossFit's annual 5-week online community competition).

Benefits of the AMRAP
Adhere to the correct training effort: Perhaps the greatest benefit of an AMRAP is that it is easier to adhere to the correct training effort—this is particularly important to novice athletes, but applies to athletes of all levels. For a novice athlete, a sprint workout can easily turn into a marathon. Take a workout like Fran for example: 21-15-9 of thrusters and pull-ups. An experienced athlete can complete this workout in less than three minutes, whereas a beginner may

take twenty. Obviously, the stimuli provided to each athlete are very different. In an AMRAP, however, 12 minutes is 12 minutes, for example. Both an advanced and novice athlete should get the same stimuli (as long as the workout is scaled properly).

Measure Progress: While you can technically measure your progress with any of the workouts in this book, I believe AMRAPs are the best way to measure improvements in work capacity. I'll often have an athlete complete a 5, 10, and 15 minute AMRAP (on different days). Six months later, they'll retest those same AMRAPs. The results will provide us with feedback on where an athlete is improving and where an athlete still needs work. For example, if an athlete was able to increase their total reps in the 15 minute AMRAP by 15% but failed to improve on the five minute AMRAP, that's likely a good indicator that they need to increase the number of workouts in that particular time domain.

Time efficiency: To maximize your performance in an AMRAP, athletes must 'tune into their bodies' to identify the pace they can keep. In the sample workout provided (12 minute AMRAP of 12 burpees, 10 butterfly sit-ups, and 8 air squats) the first question you should ask yourself in determining the proper pace is: "How hard can I work for 12 minutes?" At the end of the 12 minutes it is equally important to assess whether you went too hard or whether you were too conservative. Keep in mind that in my time analyzing athletes, I've noticed it is just as common for athletes to underestimate their work capacity as it is for them to overestimate it (going too easy versus going too hard).

AMRAP WOD 1
11 Minute AMRAP
6 Deadlifts (225/155)
8 Over-the-Bar Burpees
5 Bar Muscle-Ups

AMRAP WOD 2
16 Minute AMRAP
50 Calorie Row
50 Toes-to-Bar
40 Kettlebell Snatches, Alternating Hands (53/35)
40 Box Jumps (24/20)
30 Alternating Pistols
30 Pull-ups

AMRAP WOD 3
8 Minute AMRAP
4 Deadlifts (225/155)
10 Russian Kettlebell Swings (70/53)
5 Box Jumps (30/24)

AMRAP WOD 4
11 Minute AMRAP
6 Slamball Ground to Over-the-Shoulder (100/70)
10 Chest-to-Bar Pull-ups

AMRAP WOD 5
10 Minute AMRAP
12 Alternating In-Place Front Rack Lunges (135/95)
10 Chest-to-Bar Pull-ups
8 Over- the-Bar Burpees

AMRAP WOD 6
10 Minute AMRAP
8 Hang Power Cleans (115/80)
10 Calorie Row
12 Goblet Squat (70/53)

AMRAP WOD 7
9 Minute AMRAP
9 Thrusters (95/65)
35 Double-unders

AMRAP WOD 8
8 Minute AMRAP
16/13 Calorie Bike
10 Box Jumps (24/20)

AMRAP WOD 9
12 Minute AMRAP
25 Wall Balls (20/14)
20 Russian Kettlebell Swings (55/35)
10 Burpees

AMRAP WOD 10
11 Minute AMRAP
3 Hang Power Cleans
5 Thrusters
7 Shoulder-to-Overhead
10 Push-ups
10 Strict Pull-ups
Bar Weight: 115/80

AMRAP WOD 11
10 Minute AMRAP
3 Shoulder-to-Overhead
3 Hang Power Cleans

6 Shoulder-to-Overhead
6 Hang Power Cleans

9 Shoulder-to-Overhead
9 Hang Power Cleans
Continue this pattern, adding 3 reps to each exercise on every round.
Bar Weight: 135/95

AMRAP WOD 12
9 Minute AMRAP
20/16 Calorie Bike
15 Kettlebell Swings (70/53)
15 Toes-to-Bar

AMRAP WOD 13
9 Minute AMRAP
3 Hang Power Snatches (165/115)
6 Strict Handstand Push-ups

AMRAP WOD 14
8 Minute AMRAP
12/10 Calorie Bike
8 Slamball Over-the-Shoulder (100/70)
25-Yard Slamball Bear Hug Carry (100/70)
5 Deficit Handstand Push-ups

AMRAP WOD 15
10 Minute AMRAP
15 Overhead Squats (95/80)
30 Double-unders

AMRAP WOD 16
12 Minute AMRAP
5 Power Cleans (185/130)
10 Chest-to-Bar Pull-ups
15 Double-unders

AMRAP WOD 17
14 Minute AMRAP
4 Overhead Squats
4 Deadlifts
4 Box Jumps

6 Overhead Squats
6 Deadlifts
6 Box Jumps

8 Overhead Squats
8 Deadlifts
8 Box Jumps
Continue this pattern, adding 2 reps to each movement every round.
Bar Weight: 115/80
Box Jump Height: 24/20

AMRAP WOD 18
7 Minute AMRAP
7 Deadlifts (275/190)
5 Bar Muscle-ups

AMRAP WOD 19
10 Minute AMRAP
12 Dumbbell Squat Snatches, Alternating Hands(50/35)
10/8 Calorie Row
8 Toes-to-Bar

AMRAP WOD 20
12 Minute AMRAP
20 Kettlebell Swings (70/53)
30 Wall Balls (20/14)
10 Box Jumps (24/20)

AMRAP WOD 21
9 Minute AMRAP
10 Chest-to-Bar Pull-ups
10 Front Squats (155/110)

AMRAP WOD 22
10 Minute AMRAP
5 Snatches (115/80)
5 Over-the-Bar Burpees

AMRAP WOD 23
15 Minute AMRAP
55 Double-unders
15 Pull-ups
5 Hang Power Cleans (155/105)

AMRAP WOD 24
9 Minute AMRAP
20 Overhead Squats (95/65)
10 Bar Facing Over-the-Bar Burpees

AMRAP WOD 25
6 Minute AMRAP
21 Thrusters (95/65)
15 Toes-to-Bar

AMRAP WOD 26
10 Minute AMRAP
Max Unbroken Wall Balls (20/14)
20 Calorie Bike
Score=Total Wall Balls

AMRAP WOD 27
8 Minute AMRAP
5 Ring Muscle-Ups
8 Deadlifts (225/155)

AMRAP WOD 28
10 Minute AMRAP
15 Power Snatches (75/55)
10 Toes-to-Bar

AMRAP WOD 29
12 Minute AMRAP
400/360 Meter Row
15 Wall Balls (30/20)
10 Box Jumps (24/20)

AMRAP WOD 30
10 Minute AMRAP
15 Snatches (75/55)
10 Pull-ups

AMRAP WOD 31
12 Minutes AMRAP
20/16 Calorie Bike
15 Wall Balls (20/14)

AMRAP WOD 32
14 Minute AMRAP
60 Wall Balls (20/14)
50 Double-unders
40 GHD Sit-ups
30 Pull-ups
20 Box Jumps (24/20)

AMRAP WOD 33
10 Minute AMRAP
10 Kettlebell Swings (70/53)
10 Front Squats (115/80)

AMRAP WOD 34
12 Minute AMRAP
50 Deadlifts (185/130)
40 Toes-to-Bar
30 Wall Balls (20/14)
20 Box Jumps (24/20)
In the Remaining Time: Max Handstand Push-ups

AMRAP WOD 35
12 Minute AMRAP
25-Yard Heavy Sled Push
10 Power Snatches (95/65)

AMRAP WOD 36
7 Minute AMRAP
10 Power Snatches (75/55)
10 Chest-to-Bar Pull-ups

AMRAP WOD 37
11 Minute AMRAP
2 Power Cleans
2 Front Squats

4 Power Cleans
4 Front Squats

6 Power Cleans
6 Front Squats
Continue this pattern, adding 2 reps to each movement every round.
Bar Weight: 185/130

AMRAP WOD 38
12 Minute AMRAP
20 Wall Balls (20/14)
20/16 Calorie Row
3 15' Rope Climbs
10 Toes-to-Bar

AMRAP WOD 39
9 Minute AMRAP
10 Power Snatches (95/65)
8 Box Jumps (24/20)

AMRAP WOD 40
10 Minute AMRAP
8 Thrusters (95/65)
10/8 Calorie Bike

AMRAP WOD 41
15 Minute AMRAP
20 Wall Balls (20/14)
15 Toes-to-Bar
10 Squat Cleans (115/80)

AMRAP WOD 42
8 Minute AMRAP
6 Power Cleans (225/155)
8 Box Jumps (24/20)
10 Chest-to-Bar Pull-ups

AMRAP WOD 43
15 Minute AMRAP
10 Double Russian Kettlebell Swings (30/20)*
12 Toes-to-Bar
14 Thrusters (95/65)
16 Double-unders
*One kettlebell in each hand.

AMRAP WOD 44
15 Minute AMRAP
50 Double-unders
40 Chest-to-Bar Pull-ups
35 Wall Balls (20/14)
30 Toes-to-Bar
25 Hang Snatches (95/65)

AMRAP WOD 45
9 Minute AMRAP
3 Deadlifts
3 Box Jumps

6 Deadlifts
6 Box Jumps

9 Deadlifts
9 Box Jumps
Continue this pattern, adding 3 reps to each movement every round.
Bar Weight: 225/155
Box Jump Height: 24/20

AMRAP WOD 46
9 Minute AMRAP
12 Overhead Squats (95/65)
10 Russian Kettlebell Swings (70/53)

AMRAP WOD 47
12 Minute AMRAP
10 Overhead Squats (115/80)
10 Box Jumps (30/24)
3 15' Rope Climbs

CHAPTER 4
FOR TIME

To understand the benefits of *for time* workouts, we need to first understand the difference between time priority and task priority workouts. A time priority workout is a workout with a set amount of time. An AMRAP, where the workout time is fixed, is an example of this. A task priority workout is a workout with a set number of rounds and reps. All the workouts in this chapter are task priority workouts (for time)—that includes 'for time' couplets and triplets that were not included in previous chapters. While both types of workouts have their advantages, science—and personal experience—suggest that because athletes process time and distance differently, they tend to go harder on task priority tasks.

Inspired by a study by published in *Medicine & Science in Sports and Exercise*, to test this theory I had 14 athletes complete the following workout: 3 rounds of a 200-meter row, 8 burpee box jumps, and 8 toes-to-bar. The next day athletes were divided into two groups—seven athletes repeated the same workout while the other seven worked out for the time it took them to finish the WOD the previous day. In the first group, four athletes improved their time, one remained the same, and two finished on average 2.5 seconds slower. Similar to the study published in *Medicine & Science in Sports and Exercise*, on average the second group completed fewer reps than they did on the original workout. In summary, athletes performed better when the workout was for time versus for max reps.

As you'll likely find when you begin to tackle the workouts in this chapter, *for time* workouts allow you to see the finish line—the greater the effort you give, the faster you'll finish. In a time priority task like AMRAPs, the more effort you give, the more reps you'll accumulate, but the workout length remains the same, leading you to prioritize pace over intensity.

Other Benefits of *For Time* workouts
Holds you accountable. There's a popular phrase often said about *for time* workouts: "The clock will not save you". What this means is while you can give a minimum effort on an AMRAP and still finish (however bad your score may be), the same cannot be said about a workout for time. The nature of a task oriented workout means that you must work until you complete every round and rep that was written. Giving less effort than you should only means you'll be working for a longer time.

Increases competition. Visually, it's often easier to compete with another athlete in a task oriented workout than it is a time oriented workout. In a time oriented workout like an AMRAP, every athlete will finish at exactly the same time—at the end of the AMRAP. On the other hand, in a workout for time, it's much easier to see how ahead or behind you are of other athletes and exactly when each athlete finishes the WOD. Taken advantage of correctly, the extra boost this competition provides can do wonders for your performance and overall fitness level.

FOR TIME WOD 1
3 Rounds
10 Power Snatches
20/16 Calorie Row
15 Thrusters
10/8 Calorie Bike
Bar Weight: 95/65

FOR TIME WOD 2
50 Strict Presses
50 Pull-ups
50 Handstand Push-ups
10/8 Calorie Row on Every Break*
*Example: If you perform 15 strict presses and put the bar down, you must row 10/8 calories before you continue your presses. You do not have to row when transitioning between movements.
Bar Weight: 45/35

FOR TIME WOD 3
4 Rounds
20 Calorie Row
15 Wall Balls (30/20)
10 Kettlebell Swings (70/53)
20 Kettlebell In-Place Overhead Lunges (40/25)*
Use only one kettlebell.

FOR TIME WOD 4
1500 Meter Row
65 Thrusters (45/35)
45 Toes-to-Bar

FOR TIME WOD 5
8 Rounds
10 Wall Balls (30/20)
8 Alternating Dumbbell Squat Snatches (55/35)
6 Chest-to-bar pull-ups
*500 Meter Row Buy-in and Buy-out

FOR TIME WOD 6
3 Rounds
12 Alternating In-Place Front Rack Lunges (135/95)
10 Chest-to-Bar Pull-ups
8 Over-the-Bar Burpees

-rest 5 minutes-

3 Rounds
20 Kettlebell Swings (55/35)
10 Box Jumps

FOR TIME WOD 7
30 Calorie Row
25 Wall Balls
2 Complexes of 5 Deadlifts, 4 Hang Cleans, 3 Front Squat, 2 Jerks
10 Box Jumps (30/24)

20 Calorie Row
15 Wall Balls
2 Complexes of 5 Deadlifts, 4 Hang Cleans, 3 Front Squat, 2 Jerks
5 Box Jumps (30/24)
*Once you begin a complex, you may not put the bar down.
Bar Weight: 135/95
Wall Ball: 20/14

FOR TIME WOD 8
35 Toes-to-Bar
70 Wall Balls (20/14)
35 Toes-to –Bar

FOR TIME WOD 9
20/18 Calorie Row
20 Power Cleans
20 Handstand Push-ups

15/13 Calorie Row
15 Power Cleans
15 Handstand Push-ups

10/8 Calorie Row
10 Power Cleans
10 Handstand Push-ups
Bar Weight: (135/95)

FOR TIME WOD 10
30 Wall Balls (20/14)
8 Box Jumps

30 Push-ups
8 Box Jumps

30 Toes-to-Bar
8 Box Jumps

30 Ring Dips
8 Box Jumps
Box Jump Height: 24/20

FOR TIME WOD 11
100 Russian Kettlebell Swings (70/53)

FOR TIME WOD 12
12-9-6
Shoulder-to-Overhead (155/110)
Burpee Box Jump Overs (24/20)

-straight into-

100 Double-unders
50 Kettlebell Swings (70/53)
30 Toes-to-bar
100 Double-unders

FOR TIME WOD 13
500/450 Meter Row
21 Deadlifts
15 Toes-to-Bar
9 Muscle-ups

500/450 Meter Row
15 Deadlifts
15 Toes-to-Bar
6 Muscle-ups

500/450 Meter Row
9 Deadlifts
15 Toes-to-Bar
3 Muscle-ups
Bar Weight: 225/155

FOR TIME WOD 14
15-9-6
Calorie Bike
Box Jump Overs (24/20)

-straight into-

21 Calorie Row
4 15' Rope Climb

15 Calorie Row
3 15' Rope Climb

9 Calorie Row
2 15' Rope Climb

FOR TIME WOD 15
21 Deadlifts
25-Yard Farmers Carry
21 Kettlebell Thrusters

15 Deadlifts
25-Yard Farmers Carry
15 Kettlebell Thrusters*

9 Deadlifts
25-Yard Farmers Carry
9 Kettlebell Thrusters
Deadlift Weight: 225/155
Kettlebell Weight: 53/35
*Farmers Carry Weight: 155/110**
*Use two kettlebells for the thrusters.
*If you don't have Farmer Carry bars, use two heavy kettlebells.

FOR TIME WOD 16

500/450 Meter Row
50 Wall Balls (20/14)

500/450 Meter Row
50 Double-unders

500/450 Meter Row
50 Kettlebell Swings (53/35)

FOR TIME WOD 17

5 Thrusters (155/105)
4 Weighted Pull-Ups

4 Thrusters (175/120)
6 Weighted Pull-Ups

3 Thrusters (195/135)
8 Weighted Pull-Ups

2 Thrusters (215/150)
10 Weighted Pull-Ups

1 Thruster (235/165)
12 Weighted Pull-Ups
Pull-up weight should be as heavy as possible while maintaining good form.

FOR TIME WOD 18

20 Clean + Jerks
30 Calorie Row
40 Russian Kettlebell Swings (70/53)
20 Calorie Row
10 Snatches
Bar Weight: 135/95

FOR TIME WOD 19

20-Yard Heavy Sled Push
3 15' Rope Climbs
10 Squat Snatches

20-Yard Heavy Sled Push
2 15' Rope Climbs
8 Squat Snatches

20-Yard Heavy Sled Push
1 15' Rope Climb
6 Squat Snatches
Bar Weight: 135/95

FOR TIME WOD 20

21-15-9
Thrusters (95/65)
Calorie Bike
Chest-to-Bar Pull-ups
Toes-to-Bar

FOR TIME WOD 21

2 Rounds
20-Yard Moderate Weight Sled Push
2 15' Rope Climbs
8 Cleans + Jerks (135/95)
10 Burpee Box Jumps (30/24)
400 Meter Run
25 Double-unders

FOR TIME WOD 22
1000 Meter Row
21 Power Cleans
21 Barbell Rows

800 Meter Row
15 Power Cleans
15 Barbell Rows

500 Meter Row
9 Power Cleans
9 Barbell Rows

250 Meter Row
3 Power Cleans
3 Barbell Rows
Bar Weight: 135/95

FOR TIME WOD 23
3 Rounds
400 Meter Run
25-Yard Overhead Dumbbell Lunges (50/35)*
20 GHD Sit-ups
15 Calorie Bike
5 Man Makers (50/35)
*One dumbbell in each hand.

FOR TIME WOD 24
30 Snatches
30 Pull-ups
15 Snatches
15 Pull-ups
Bar Weight: 115/80

FOR TIME WOD 25
15-9-6
Dumbbell Thrusters* (50/35)
Chest-to-Bar Pull-ups
Calorie Row
Burpees
One dumbbell in each hand.

FOR TIME WOD 26
6 Squat Cleans
12 Bar Facing Over-the-Bar Burpees
24 Pull-ups
12 Bar Facing Over-the-Bar Burpees
6 Squat Cleans
Bar Weight: 255/1175

FOR TIME WOD 27
21 Deadlifts (225/155)
42/35 Calorie Row

15 Cleans (185/130)
30/25 Calorie Row

9 Squat Snatches (135/95)
18/14 Calorie Row

FOR TIME WOD 28
3 Rounds
21 Russian Kettlebell Swings (70/53)
18 Wall Balls (20/14)
15 Chest-to-Bar Pull-ups
12 Burpees

FOR TIME WOD 29
2 Rounds
300 Meter Row
20 Burpees

-straight into-

2 Rounds
500 Meter Row
30 Air Squats

-straight into-

1 Round
700 Meter Row
20 Burpees

-straight into-

1 Round
1000 Meter Row
30 Air Squats

FOR TIME WOD 30
4 Rounds
12 Overhead Squats (95/65)
10 Calorie Bike
8 Burpees
6 Bar Muscle-ups

FOR TIME WOD 31
3 Rounds
20-Yard Front Rack Lunges (165/115)
15 Burpee Box Jump Overs (24/20)
20 Wall Balls (30/20)
15 Chest-to-Bar Pull-ups

FOR TIME WOD 32

30 Calorie Row
30 Pull-ups

25 Calorie Row
25 Handstand Push-ups

20 Calorie Row
20 Box Jumps (30/20)

15 Calorie Row
15 Ring Muscle-ups

10 Calorie Row
25-Yard Handstand Walk

FOR TIME WOD 33

3 Rounds
21 Russian Kettlebell Swings (70/53)
15 Box Jumps (24/20)
9 Clean + Jerks (155/110)
Before Every Round Complete:
25-Yard Light Sled Push
25-Yard Light Sled Pull

FOR TIME WOD 34

21 Thrusters
42 Calorie Row

15 Squat Cleans
30 Calorie Row

9 Squat Snatches
18 Calorie Row
Bar Weight: 135/95

FOR TIME WOD 35
30 Box Jumps (24/20)
30 Overhead Squats (115/80)
30 Toes-to-Bar
30 Over-the-Bar Burpees

FOR TIME WOD 36
3 Rounds
10 Snatches (95/65)
12 Toes-to-Bar
12 Russian Kettlebell Swings (70/53)
14 Wall Balls (20/14)

FOR TIME WOD 37
15-9-6
Pistols, Alternating
Bar Muscle-ups
Toes-to-Bar
Hang Snatches (135/95)

FOR TIME WOD 38
2 Rounds
30 Overhead Squats
25 Pull-ups
20 Thrusters
15 Toes-to-Bar
Bar Weight: 115/80

FOR TIME WOD 39
21-15-9
Push Presses
GHD Sit-ups
In-place Alternating Overhead Lunges
Burpees
Bar Weight: 95/65

FOR TIME WOD 40
8 Rounds
4 Deadlifts (275/190)
4 Over-the-Bar Burpees
4 Bar Muscle-Ups
4 Man Makers (30/20)

FOR TIME WOD 41
2 Rounds
30 Overhead Squats
25 Pull-ups
20 Thrusters
15 Toes-to-Bar
Bar Weight: 115/80

FOR TIME WOD 42
2000 Meter Row
50 Wall Balls (20/14)
50 Pull-ups
50 Kettlebell Swings (53/35)

FOR TIME WOD 43
5 Squat Cleans (225/155)
40 Handstand Push-ups

4 Squat Cleans (235/165)
40 Chest-to-Bar Pull-ups

3 Squat Cleans (245/170)
40 Toes-to-Bar

2 Squat Cleans (255/175)
40 Push-ups

FOR TIME WOD 44
4 Rounds
21 Sumo Deadlift High Pulls (70/53)
18 Wall Balls (20/14)
15 Pull-ups
12 Burpees

FOR TIME WOD 45
27 Overhead Squats
21 Calorie Row
15 Bar Muscle-Ups
9 Squat Snatches
Bar Weight: 115/80

FOR TIME WOD 46
3 Rounds
20 Wall Balls (20/14)
15 Butterfly Sit-ups with Med Ball (20/14)
10 Box Jumps (24/20)
*Buy-In/Buy-Out: 400 Meter Run With Med Ball (20/14)

FOR TIME WOD 47

1000 Meter Row
10 Burpees
10 Ring Dips
20 Thrusters

700 Meter Row
10 Burpees
10 Ring Dips
20 Thrusters

400 Meter Row
10 Burpees
10 Ring Dips
20 Thrusters
Thruster Weight: 45/35

CHAPTER 5
INTERVALS

Interval workouts involve short periods of work followed by a recovery period (this can mean complete rest or less intense work). This is one of my preferred forms of training as studies have shown the training effects to be superior to continuous exercise for the same period of time. Of course, like anything else, interval training is only effective when applied correctly. In this case, it is important that athletes apply equal importance to both components of the workout: the work period *and* the recovery period. As such, scaling this type of workout will often be different than any other in this book.

One type of interval structure used throughout this chapter is EMOMs. EMOM stands for Every Minute On the Minute. During an EMOM, an athlete performs a set number of reps of a given movement at the beginning of each minute. The athlete has a minute to complete the task; once completed, they have whatever time is left of the minute to rest. The next work period begins at the top of the following minute. *Let's look at some sample EMOMs:*

Interval WOD
10 Minute EMOM
8 Burpees

This is as simple as an EMOM gets. At the beginning of every minute, you'll perform 8 burpees. If you finish those burpees in 35 seconds, you'll have 25 seconds to rest before starting the next set of burpees.

How to scale: For any EMOM, you'll want to scale the number of reps so that you can finish with sufficient time to rest and recover for the next minute. Let's assume it takes you a full minute to complete the eight burpees. Unfortunately, this doesn't leave you any rest time. Remember, the recovery period is just as important as the work period. Seven reps will allow you to finish the first minute of burpees in just over 50 seconds. Is less than ten seconds of rest enough time to recover so that you can finish all 10 rounds of the EMOM consistently? Probably not. Six reps will have you finish in just over 40 seconds. Will that give you enough recovery time? Understand that scaling isn't a science. In our example, 5-6 reps will probably be the magic number. If you decide to go with six burpees and find that you're running out of time by the fourth or fifth round, scale down to five (or four) reps for the remainder of the workout.

Throughout the chapter you're going to see several variations of EMOMs:

More than one movement per minute. An EMOM may require you to complete two or three movements every minute; for example, an eight minute EMOM of 10 overhead squats (95/65)* and 24 double-unders. When scaling a workout like this, try to scale both movements evenly. For example, instead of trying to move fast on the overhead squats and scaling the weight to 45/15 while keeping the 24 double-unders the same, you can scale more evenly by dropping the overhead squats to 65/45 and reducing the double-unders to 15 reps. Again, remember that scaling a workout is an art, not a science—you'll get better at it with time.

*In an EMOM, scale non-weight bearing movements by reps (burpees, double-unders, pull-ups, etc.). When scaling weight bearing movements (overhead squats, thrusters, power cleans, etc.) scale by weight.

Rx 10 Minute EMOM 10 Overhead Squats (95/65) 24 Double-unders	Scaling Option 1* 10 Minute EMOM 10 Overhead Squats (45/15) 24 Double-unders *Only scales the squats	Scaling Option 2* 10 Minute EMOM 10 Overhead Squats (65/45) 18 Double-unders *Scales both movements

A different movement every minute. Many of the workouts throughout this chapter will actually have you do a different movement every minute. Let's take a look at a sample workout and how to read it:

16 Minute EMOM
M1: 12 Handstand Push-ups
M2: 10 Power Cleans (155/110)
M3: 8 Chest-to-Bar Pull-ups
M4: Rest

This 16-minute EMOM will have you complete 12 handstand push-ups the first minute, 10 power cleans the second, 8 chest-to-bar pull-ups the third, and the fourth minute will be used to rest (despite the rest time provided on the fourth minute, you should still have built-in rest periods every minute). After the fourth minute, complete the intervals again. You'll do this a total of four times until the 16 minutes are complete (4x4=16).

Scale this workout just like we scaled the previous two examples. You want to give yourself enough time to rest and recover between movements so you can consistently finish each work period.

INTERVAL WOD 1
<u>15 Minute Interval AMRAP</u>
6 Minute AMRAP
30/20 Calorie Bike
500/450 Meter Row
Max Squat Snatches In The Remaining Time (135/95)

-rest 3 minutes-

6 Minute AMRAP
20/15 Calorie Bike
400/360 Meter Row
Max Squat Snatches In The Remaining Time (135/95)

INTERVAL WOD 2
21 Calorie Bike
21 Thrusters (95/65)

-rest 2 minutes-

15 Calorie Bike
15 Thrusters (115/80)

-rest 1.5 minutes-

9 Calorie Bike
9 Thrusters (135/95)

INTERVAL WOD 3
25 Minute EMOM
M1: 10 Power Snatches (115/80)
M2: 250/220 Meter Row
M3: 12 Handstand Push-ups
M4: 14 Alternating Pistols
M5: Rest

INTERVAL WOD 4
15 Minute Interval AMRAP
6 Minute AMRAP
10 Power Snatches (95/65)
8 Over-the-Bar Burpees
6 Box Jumps (24/20)

-rest 3 minutes-

6 Minute AMRAP
10 Power Cleans (115/80)
8 Over-the-Bar Burpees
6 Box Jumps (24/20)

INTERVAL WOD 5
8 Minute EMOM
10 Overhead Squats (95/65)
24 Double-unders

INTERVAL WOD 6
24 Minute EMOM
M1: 12/10 Calorie Bike
M2: 25-Yard Moderate Sled Pull (135/90)
M3: 15 Wall Balls (24/20)
M4: 25-Yard Moderate Sled Pull (135/90)

INTERVAL WOD 7
Every 2 Minutes for 14 Minutes
8 Deadlifts (275/190)
6 Over-the-Bar Burpees
4 Pistols (Per Leg)

INTERVAL WOD 8
12 Minute EMOM
M1: 12/10 Calorie Row
M2: 3 Squat Snatches (155/110)
M3: 30 Second L-Sit Hold (on parallettes)

INTERVAL WOD 9
Every 2 Minutes for 16 Minutes
10 Pull-ups
10 Toes-to-Bar
Max Calorie Row in the remaining time
Rest the last 30 seconds of every round.

INTERVAL WOD 10
9 Minute EMOM
M1: 2 15' Rope Climbs
M2: 5 Power Cleans (135/95)
M3: 12/8 Calorie Bike

INTERVAL WOD 11
15 Minute EMOM
M1: 5 Power Snatches
M2: 10 Barbell Back Rows
M3: 6 Push-ups + 6 Ring Dips
Bar Weight: 60% of your max snatch

INTERVAL WOD 12
5 Rounds
500/450 Meter Row
10 Fronts Squats @ 60% of Your Max*
Rest 2 minutes between rounds.
Front squats off the rack.

INTERVAL WOD 13
20 Clean + Jerks (135/95)

-rest 2 minutes-

30 Push-ups
30 Ring Dips

-rest 2 minutes-

200 Double-unders

-rest 2 minutes-

40/32 Calorie Bike

INTERVAL WOD 14
Every 5 Minutes for 20 Minutes
10 Box Jumps (24/20)
12 Burpees
14 Toes-to-Bar
14/10 Calorie Bike

INTERVAL WOD 15
18 Minute EMOM
M0-2: 10 Power Clean + Jerks (@ 60% of Max)
M2-3: 10 Strict Weighted Pull-ups (As heavy as possible)
M3-4: 10 Push-ups + 8 Ring Dips
M4-6: rest

INTERVAL WOD 16
15 Minute EMOM
M1: 5 Strict Handstand Push-ups + 7 Kipping Handstand Push-ups
M2: 12 Muscle Snatches (75/55)
M3: Rest

INTERVAL WOD 17
18 Minute EMOM
M1: 250/220 Meter Row
M2: 10 Back Hypers
M3: 10 Strict Presses (95/65)

INTERVAL WOD 18
12 Minute EMOM
M1: 40 Double-unders
M2: 250/220 Meter Row
M3: 16 Thrusters (45/35)

INTERVAL WOD 19
11 Minute Interval EMOM
3 Minute EMOM
15 Power Snatches (75/50)
15 Air Squats

-rest 1 minute-

3 Minute EMOM
9 Power Snatches (95/65)
9 Air Squats

-rest 1 minute-

3 Minute EMOM
15 Power Snatches (75/50)
9 Air Squats

INTERVAL WOD 20
12 Minute EMOM
M1: Max Strict Pull-ups
M2: Max Clean + Jerks (135/95)
M3: Rest

INTERVAL WOD 21
10 Minute EMOM
M1: 250/220 Meter Row
M2: 15 Over-the-Row Burpees

INTERVAL WOD 22
4 Rounds
20-Yard Back Rack Lunges (135/95)
20 Russian Kettlebell Swings (53/35)
Rest 1 minute between rounds.

INTERVAL WOD 23
11 Minute EMOM
M1: 21 Russian Kettlebell Swings
M2: 15 Russian Kettlebell Swings
M3: 9 Russian Kettlebell Swings
M4: Rest
M5: 21 Snatches
M6: 15 Snatches
M7: 9 Snatches
M8: Rest
M9: 15 GHD Sit-ups + 5 Russian Kettlebell Swings
M10: 10 GHD Sit-ups + 10 Russian Kettlebell Swings
M11: 5 GHD Sit-ups + 15 Russian Kettlebell Swings
Kettlebell Weight: 75/53
Bar Weight: 75/55

INTERVAL WOD 24
10 Minute EMOM
8 Wall Balls (20/14)
7 Burpees

INTERVAL WOD 25
4 Rounds
21 Thrusters (95/65)
21 Calorie Row
21 Kettlebell Swings (53/35)
Rest 1.5 minutes between rounds.

INTERVAL WOD 26
16 Minute EMOM
M1: 12 Handstand Push-ups
M2: 10 Power Cleans (155/110)
M3: 8 Chest-to-Bar Pull-ups
M4: Rest

INTERVAL WOD 27
5 Rounds
5 Thrusters (135/95)
10/8 Calorie Bike

-rest 3 minutes-

4 Rounds
10 Thrusters (95/65)
10 Toes-to-Bar

-rest 3 minutes-

3 Rounds
20 Thrusters (45/35)
10/8 Calorie Bike
10 Toes-to-Bar

INTERVAL WOD 28
24 Minute EMOM
M1: 250/225 Meter Row
M2: 12 Russian Kettlebell Swings (53/35)
M3: 12 Toes-to-Bar
M4: 20 Thrusters (45/35)

INTERVAL WOD 29
Every 2 Minutes for 12 Minutes
M0-2: 15 Thrusters (95/65)
M2-4: 9 Thrusters (115/80)
M4-6: 15 Thrusters (95/65)
M6-8: 6 Thrusters (135/95)
M8-10: 15 Thrusters (95/65)
M10-12: 3 Thrusters (165/115)

INTERVAL WOD 30
Every 1.5 Minutes for 15 Minutes
12 Push Jerks (115/80)
10 Kettlebell Sumo Deadlift High Pulls (70/53)

INTERVAL WOD 31
24 Minute EMOM
M1: 10 Dumbbell Squat Snatches, Alternating Hands (50/35)
M2: 15 GHD Sit-ups
M3: 20 Bar Thrusters (45/35)
M4: 12/8 Calorie Bike

INTERVAL WOD 32
Every 2 Minutes For 16 Minutes
M0-2: 30 Double-unders
M2-4: 5 Clean + Jerks (185/130)
M4-6: 12 Chest-to-Bar Pull-Ups or 6 Ring Muscle-Ups
M6-8: 10 Pistols + 8 Burpees

INTERVAL WOD 33
50 Wall Balls (20/14)
100 Double-unders

-rest 1 minute-

50 Kettlebell Swings (70/53)
25 Burpees

-rest 1 minute-

50 Handstand Push-ups
100 Double-unders

-rest 1 minute-

50 Thrusters (45/35)
25 Burpees

-rest 1 minute-

50 Calorie Bike
100 Double-unders

-rest 1 minute-

50 GHD Sit-ups
25 Burpees

INTERVAL WOD 34
Every 2 Minutes For 24 Minutes
8 Thrusters
8 In-Place Overhead Lunges
5 Over-the-Bar Burpees
Bar Weight: 95/65

INTERVAL WOD 35
8 Minute AMRAP
20/16 Calorie Bike
10 Over-the-Parallette Burpees

-rest 3 minutes-

6 Minute AMRAP
16/12 Calorie Bike
8 Over-the-Parallette Burpees

-rest 2 minutes-

4 Minute AMRAP
12/10 Calorie Bike
6 Over-the-Parallette Burpees

INTERVAL WOD 36
15 Minute EMOM
M1: 21 Thrusters
M2: 10 Over-the-Parallette Burpees
M3: 15 Squat Snatches
M4: 10 Over-the-Parallette Burpees
M5: 9 Complexes of 1 Power Clean + 1 Hang Squat Clean
M6: 10 Over-the-Parallette Burpees
M6-9: Rest
M9-15: Repeat Part 1
Bar Weight: 95/65

INTERVAL WOD 37
Every 2 Minutes For 24 Minutes
M0-2: 20/16 Calorie Bike + 10 Burpees
M2-4: 25-Yard Heavy Sled Push + 1 Legless Rope Climb

INTERVAL WOD 38
3 Rounds
15 Power Cleans (155/110)
15 Box Jumps (24/20)
15 Chest-to-Bar
15 Wall Balls (30/20)
Rest 1.5 minute between rounds.

INTERVAL WOD 39
21 Minute EMOM
M1: 300/250 Meter Row
M2: 4 Man Makers (40/30)
M3: 12 Chest-to-Bar Pull-ups

INTERVAL WOD 40
1 Round
60 Wall Balls (20/14)
30 Power Cleans (135/95)

-rest 2 minutes-

2 Rounds
10 Squat Snatches (135/95)
40 Double-unders

-rest 2 minutes-

3 Rounds
15 Wall Balls (20/14)
30 Double-unders

INTERVAL WOD 41
15 Minute EMOM
5 Burpees
1 Clean +Jerk (235/165)

INTERVAL WOD 42
16 Minute Interval AMRAP
4 Minute AMRAP (Minutes 0-4)
3 Power Cleans
3 Shoulder-to-Overhead
3 Front Squats

4 Minute AMRAP (Minutes 4-8)
6 Wall Balls
6 Box Jumps
6 Toes To Bar

4 Minute AMRAP (Minutes 8-12)
3 Power Cleans
3 Shoulder-to-Overhead
3 Front Squats

4 Minute AMRAP (Minutes 12-16)
6 Wall Balls
6 Box Jumps
6 Toes-to-Bar
Bar Weight: 135/95
Wall Balls: 20/14
Box Jump: 24/20

INTERVAL WOD 43
30 Calorie Bike
600 Meter Run
500 Meter Row

-rest 2 minutes-

20 Calorie Bike
400 Meter Run
400 Meter Row

-rest 1.5 minutes-

10 Calorie Bike
200 Meter Run
300 Meter Row

-rest 1 minute-

20 Calorie Bike
400 Meter Run
400 Meter Row

-rest 1.5 minutes-

30 Calorie Bike
600 Meter Run
500 Meter Row

INTERVAL WOD 44
18 Minute EMOM
M1: 8 Thrusters (135/95)
M2: 10 Box Jumps (20/14)
M3: 300/270m Row

INTERVAL WOD 45

12 Deadlifts (95/65)
11 Power Cleans (95/65)

-rest 1 minute-

11 Deadlifts (115/80)
10 Power Cleans (115/80)

-rest 1 minute-

10 Deadlifts (135/95)
9 Power Cleans (135/95)

-rest 1 minute-

9 Deadlifts (155/110)
8 Power Cleans (155/110)

-rest 1 minute-

8 Deadlifts (175/120)
7 Power Cleans (175/120)

-rest 1 minute-

7 Deadlifts (195/135)
6 Power Cleans (195/135)

-rest 1 minute-

6 Deadlifts (215/150)
5 Power Cleans (215/150)

-rest 1 minute-

5 Deadlifts (235/165)
4 Power Cleans (235/165)

INTERVAL WOD 46

40 Thrusters
30 Calorie Row
40 Toes-to-Bar
30 Calorie Row

-rest 2 minutes-

30 Thrusters
20 Calorie Row
30 Toes-to-Bar
20 Calorie Row

-rest 1.5 minutes-

20 Thrusters
10 Calorie Row
20 Toes-to-Bar
10 Calorie Row
Thrusters: 95/65

CHAPTER 6
GYMNASTICS

A focus on gymnastics is arguably the most underappreciated aspect of functional fitness training. However, consistently incorporating gymnastics in, body awareness, flexibility and mobility, and one of the most underrated components of a great athlete—patience. Furthermore, the reality is that a heavy majority of all WODs feature some gymnastics element. I strongly believe that developing efficient movements in this is area will give most athletes the biggest return in improved performances in workouts.

The following chapter includes 29 gymnastic intensive workouts. More than any of the other workouts in this book, there's a trade-off between keeping intensity high and using the WODs to focus on proper movement and skill development. If we look at Gymnastics Workout 29 for example:

6 Minute EMOM
10 Chest-to-Bar Pull-ups

If you're not proficient enough at chest-to-bar pull-ups to perform them in a WOD, what foundational movement can you replace them with that will help get you there? Strict pull ups, ring rows, negatives? What if you are proficient enough to do the workout as prescribed? Once completed, examine where your chest-to-bar pull-ups broke down, for example. If your form broke down on the third round, was it because of a lack of strength or skill? More than likely, it's a combination of the two. However, this is where your patience can lead our investigation in the right direction. Did your form break down because of a lack of strength or did your strength break down because your movements were inefficient? Whatever the case, take the information acquired from this, and every other gymnastics workout, and use it to go back to the foundations that are limiting you.

GYMNASTICS WOD 1
4 Rounds
5 Bar Muscle-ups
15 Handstand Push-ups

GYMNASTICS WOD 2
3 Rounds
25-Yard Handstand Walk
20 Push-ups
15 Ring Dips

GYMNASTICS WOD 3
<u>16 Minute Interval EMOM</u>
4 Minute EMOM
10 Toes-to-Bar

4 Minute EMOM
10 Chest-to-Bar Pull-ups

4 Minute EMOM
10 Ring Dips

4 Minute EMOM
10 Handstand Push-ups

GYMNASTICS WOD 4
4 Rounds
5 Strict Pull-ups
5 Kipping or Butterfly Pull-ups
5 Chest-to-Bar Pull-ups
5 Bar Muscle-ups
Rest 1.5 minutes between rounds.

GYMNASTICS WOD 5
5 Minute EMOM
5 Ring Muscle-ups

GYMNASTICS WOD 6
15 Minute AMRAP
12 Burpees
6 Ring Muscle-ups

GYMNASTICS WOD 7
5 Rounds
45 Double-unders
15 Handstand Push-ups

GYMNASTICS WOD 8
50 Ring Push-ups
50 Strict Pull-ups
50 Weighted Ringed Dips (20/15)

GYMNASTICS WOD 9
100 Alternating Weighted Pistols (35/25)

GYMNASTICS WOD 10
4 Rounds
10 Chest-to-Bar Pull-ups
12 Alternating Pistols

GYMNASTICS WOD 11
4 Rounds
5 Bar Muscle-ups
5 Deficit Handstand Push-up
5 Ring Push-ups

GYMNASTICS WOD 12
15-9-6
Strict Handstand Push-ups
Bar Muscle-ups

GYMNASTICS WOD 13
AMRAP*
5 Unbroken Ring Muscle-ups
10 GHD Sit-ups
Rest 1 Minute Between Rounds.
*Continue the AMRAP until you can no longer complete the 5 unbroken muscle-ups.

GYMNASTICS WOD 14
40 Toes-to-bar
2 15' Rope Climbs
40 Alternating Pistols
4 15' Rope Climbs
40 Chest-to-Bar Pull-ups
6 15' Rope Climbs

GYMNASTICS WOD 15
3 Rounds
8 Bar Muscle-ups
20-Yard Handstand Walk

GYMNASTICS WOD 16
For Time
60 Handstand Push-ups
50 Pull-ups
10 15' Rope Climbs

GYMNASTICS WOD 17
For Time
50 GHD Sit-ups
75 Toes-to-Bar
100 Double-unders

GYMNASTICS WOD 18
21-15-9
Handstand Push-ups
Pistols, Alternating
Bar Muscle-ups

GYMNASTICS WOD 19
18 Minute EMOM
M1: 4 Ring Muscle-ups
M2: 30 Second Handstand Hold Against Wall
M3: 30 Double-unders

GYMNASTICS WOD 20
4 Rounds
8 3' Burpees Broad Jumps
10 Strict Handstand Push-ups
12 Toes-to-Bar

GYMNASTICS WOD 21
15 Minute AMRAP
3 15' Legless Rope Climbs
13 Burpee Pull-ups

GYMNASTICS WOD 22
12 Minute AMRAP
4 Strict Ring Muscle-ups
25-Yard Handstand Walk

GYMNASTICS WOD 23
3 Rounds
20 GHD Sit-ups
20 Handstand Push-ups
20 Alternating Pistols (40/30)

GYMNASTICS WOD 24
Every 2 Minutes For 20 Minutes
1 15' Legless Rope Climbs
3 Complexes of: 5 Toes-to-Bar, 5 Chest-to-Bar Pull-ups*
Cannot come off the bar mid complex. Need to be unbroken. Can come off the bar between complexes if necessary.

GYMNASTICS WOD 25
16 Minute EMOM
M1: 12 Handstand Push-ups
M2: 12 Chest-to-Bar Pull-ups
M3: 12 Burpees
M4: 40 Double-unders

GYMNASTICS WOD 26
3 Rounds
10 Ring Muscle-ups
3 15' Rope Climbs

GYMNASTICS WOD 27
8 Minute AMRAP
20 Pull-ups
10 Burpees
20 Toes-to-Bar
10 Burpees

GYMNASTICS WOD 28
5 Minute EMOM
20 Second L-Sit Hold on Parallettes
40 Second Rest

GYMNASTICS WOD 29
6 Minute EMOM
10 Chest-to-Bar Pull-ups

CHAPTER 7
BODYWEIGHT

Bodyweight exercises, just like working out with a barbell or kettlebell, affords numerous benefits including improved overall endurance, body awareness, heart health, the health of joints and bones, and helping to build lean body mass. These benefits are accentuated when bodyweight workouts are incorporated in an overall fitness plan. Performing air squats, for example, can help detect improper movement patterns that may not be as easily detectable when squatting heavy loads. This isn't to say that air squats are only necessary because they improve squatting with weight; in fact, air squats are an excellent exercise to build muscle, strength, and improve endurance. Incorporating sprints or broad jumps can help develop the explosiveness needed for lifts like the snatch and clean and jerk. Plank holds and V-ups can help you build the core strength needed for more weight bearing activities—and other more general life activities like avoiding back pain and carrying groceries. The list goes on!

Bodyweight WODs are also great because you can do them almost anywhere; although you'll need some equipment when the workout calls for movements like pull-ups or ring dips, for example. The point is, there's no need for your fitness to suffer just because can't make it to the gym. Take Bodyweight WOD 20:

6 Rounds
10 Burpees
10 Jumping Air Squats
100 Meter Sprint
Buy-in/Buy-out: Accumulate 1 Minute of Plank Holds

Bodyweight WOD 20 is a challenging workout that will, among other things, work your cardiovascular endurance, explosiveness, core, and quads—and you don't need any special equipment to perform it.

BODYWEIGHT WOD 1
100 Air Squats
80 Butterfly Sit-ups
60 Alternating Jumping Lunges
40 Push-ups
20 Burpees

BODYWEIGHT WOD 2
12 Minute AMRAP
20 3' Burpees Broad Jumps
15 Handstand Push-ups
10 Pull-ups

BODYWEIGHT WOD 3
400 Meter Run
30 Push-ups
30 Toes-to-Bar
30 Pull-ups
400 Meter Run
25 Push-ups
25 Toes-to-Bar
25 Pull-ups
400 Meter Run
20 Push-ups
20 Toes-to-Bar
20 Pull-ups

BODYWEIGHT WOD 4
6 Rounds
10 Back Hypers
10 Alternating Pistol

BODYWEIGHT WOD 5
4 Rounds
10 Strict Pull-ups
15 GHD Sit-ups
10 Back Hypers

BODYWEIGHT WOD 6
50 Pull-Ups
100 Air Squats
25 Pull-ups
50 Air Squats

BODYWEIGHT WOD 7
5 Rounds
50 Double-unders
10 Ring Dips
10 Ring Push-ups

BODYWEIGHT WOD 8
20 Alternating Pistols
15 Box Jumps
15 Alternating Pistols
10 Box Jumps
10 Alternating Pistols
5 Box Jumps
Box Jump Height: 24/20

BODYWEIGHT WOD 9
8 Minute AMRAP
20 Air Squats
10 Burpee Box Jumps (24/20)

BODYWEIGHT WOD 10
800 Meter Run
100 Air Squats
50 Toes To Bar
400 Meter Run

BODYWEIGHT WOD 11
14 Minute AMRAP
100 Double-unders
20 Handstand Push-ups

BODYWEIGHT WOD 12
10 Minute AMRAP
1 15' Rope Climb
4 Burpees
2 15' Rope Climbs
8 Burpees
3 15' Rope Climbs
12 Burpees
Continue this pattern, increasing 1 rope climb and 4 burpees per round.

BODYWEIGHT WOD 13
11 Minute AMRAP
12 Burpee Box Jump Overs (24/20)
10 Toes-to-Bar

BODYWEIGHT WOD 14
15 Minute AMRAP
200 Meter Run
30 Mountain Climbers
25 Jumping Air Squats
15 Burpees

BODYWEIGHT WOD 15
16 Minute EMOM
M1: Max 3' Burpee Broad Jumps
M2: Max Hand Release Push-ups
M3: Max Air Squats
M4: Max Butterfly Sit-ups

BODYWEIGHT WOD 16
6 Rounds
15 Air Squat
12 Push-ups
9 Strict Pull-ups

BODYWEIGHT WOD 17
4 Rounds
4 Legless 15' Rope Climbs
8 3' Burpee Broad Jumps
12 Handstand Push-ups

BODYWEIGHT WOD 18
16 Minute AMRAP
30 Butterfly Sit-ups
25-Yard Bear Crawl
20 Alternating Pistols

BODYWEIGHT WOD 19
4 Rounds
20-Yard Bear Crawl
20-Yards of Broad Jumps
20-Yard Crab Walk
20-Yards of Broad Jumps

BODYWEIGHT WOD 20
6 Rounds
10 Burpees
10 Jumping Air Squats
100 Meter Sprint
Buy-in/Buy-out: Accumulate 1 Minute of Plank Holds

BODYWEIGHT WOD 21
12 Minute AMRAP
14 Alternating Pistols
12 V-ups
10 Pull-ups

BODYWEIGHT WOD 22
6 Rounds
50 Double-unders
3 Rope Climbs
20 Air Squat

BODYWEIGHT WOD 23
20 Minute AMRAP
10 3' Burpee Broad Jumps
200 Meter Run

BODYWEIGHT WOD 24
4 Rounds
400 Meter Run
10 Ring Dips
12 V-ups
14 Pull-ups

BODYWEIGHT WOD 25
20 Minute AMRAP
2 15' Rope Climbs
10 Air Squats
4 15' Rope Climbs
20 Air Squats
6 15' Rope Climbs
30 Air Squats
Continue this pattern, adding 2 rope climbs and 10 air squats every round.

BODYWEIGHT WOD 26
4 Rounds
200 Meter Walking Lunge
30 V-ups
25 Push-ups
20 Pull-ups
15 Burpees

BODYWEIGHT WOD 27
100 Push-ups
100 V-ups
100 Pull-ups
*Perform 10 air squats every time you have to break.

BODYWEIGHT WOD 28
5 Rounds
16 Back Hypers
14 Push-ups
12 Jumping Air Squats

BODYWEIGHT WOD 29
14 Minute AMRAP
2 Rope Climbs
4 Ring Dips
6 Push-ups
8 Pull-ups

BODYWEIGHT WOD 30
20 Minute AMRAP
4 Air Squats
4 Push-ups
4 V-ups

6 Air Squats
6 Push-ups
6 V-ups

8 Air Squats
8 Push-ups
8 V-ups

Continue this pattern, adding 2 reps to every movement every round.

BODYWEIGHT

CHAPTER 8
PARTNER WODS

Partner WODs are a great way to add a little spice to your training. All the workouts in this chapter are designed to be completed between two people. However, if you think splitting the required work with a friend makes these workouts easier, you're in for a surprise! Some of the workouts will have you rest as your partner works while others will have both partners working at the same time. The point is, partner workouts can be just as brutal, if not more, than non-partner workouts. Having someone depend on you during a WOD often leads to you to take shorter breaks than you would in a traditional workout. Further, if your partner happens to have a glaring weakness in one of the prescribed movements, you may be left to pick up the slack.

Important Partner WOD Notes

1. **Scale to the limits of the team.** Ideally, you want to choose a partner who is at or near your fitness level. Realistically, you'll probably end up doing a partner workout at one point or another with someone of a different fitness level. It makes no sense to force someone to move a weight that is simply too heavy for them. The solution is simply to scale to the limitations of the team. Essentially, if your partner can only go so heavy on a movement, stick with that weight for the workout. Now, if you're working out with someone of the opposite sex, grab another bar and have them do their appropriate weight.

2. **Splitting up the workload.** Unless otherwise stated, partners can split up the workloads however they choose. However, unless you're in a competition setting, the goal of the workout should be to improve the fitness of *both* athletes. Therefore, proper etiquette

suggests that you split up the workload as evenly as possible.

3. Partner run. Partner runs mean just that—both partners run. I suggest you try to keep, at most, a two-foot distance between you and your partner. You don't want to be done with your 400-meter run while your partner is slugging away at the 200 meter mark. Remember, part of the added benefit of a partner WOD is that you have someone there to motivate you when the workout gets challenging.

PARTNER WOD 1
20 Squat Cleans (155/110)
20 Handstand Push-ups

16 Squat Cleans (185/130)
24 Handstand Push-ups

12 Squat Cleans (205/145)
28 Handstand Push-ups

8 Squat Cleans (225/155)
32 Handstand Push-ups

PARTNER WOD 2
60 Back Squats
50 Calorie Row
40 Pull-ups

50 Alternating In-place Back Rack Lunges
40 Calorie Row
30 Pull-ups

40 Back Squats
30 Calorie Row
20 Pull-ups
Bar Weight: 135/95

PARTNER WOD 3
50 Power Cleans
40 Burpee Box Jump Overs
400 Meter Partner Run

30 Squat Cleans
20 Burpee Box Jump Overs
400 Meter Partner Run
Bar weight: 135/95

PARTNER WOD 4
40 Thrusters
400 Partner Meter Run
40 GHD Sit-Ups

30 Thrusters
400 Partner Meter Run
30 GHD Sit-ups

20 Thrusters
400 Partner Meter Run
20 GHD Sit-ups
Bar weight: 95/65

PARTNER WOD 5
5 Rounds
15 Complexes of 1 Power Clean + 1 Hang Squat Clean + 1 Thruster (155/110)*
15 Burpee Box Jump Overs (24/20)
25 GHD Sit-ups
*Whoever begins a complex has to finish it. You may not switch mid-complex.

PARTNER WOD 6
30-25-20
Thrusters
Calorie Row
Hang Cleans
Shoulder-to-Overhead
Buy-in/Buy-out: 150 Double-unders
Bar Weight: 135/95

PARTNER WOD 7
30-25-20
Deadlifts (225/155)
Calorie Row
Synchronized 3' Burpee Broad Jumps

PARTNER WOD 8
30 Squat Cleans (165/115)
30 Over-the-Bar Bar Facing Burpees
30 Power Snatches (165/115)
30 Box Jumps (30/24)

-rest 3 minutes-

8 Alternating Rounds
5 Power Cleans (185/130)
5 Over-the-Bar Bar Facing Burpees
5 Box Jumps (30/24)

PARTNER WOD 9
100 Snatches (75/55)
8 15' Rope Climbs

90 Toes-to-Bar
6 15' Rope Climbs

80 One-Arm Dumbbell Overhead Squats (65/45)
4 15' Rope Climbs

70 Calorie Bike
2 15' Rope Climbs

PARTNER WOD 10
40-30-20-10
Deadlifts (225/155)
Calorie Bike
Before every round complete:
40-Yard Heavy Sled Push
& 4 15′ Rope Climbs

PARTNER WOD 11
50 Deadlifts (185/130)
30 Burpee Box Jump Overs

40 Deadlifts (225/155)
25 Burpee Box Jump Overs

30 Deadlifts (275/190)
20 Burpee Box Jump Overs

20 Deadlifts (315/220)
15 Burpee Box Jump Overs

10 Deadlifts (365/255)
10 Burpee Box Jump Overs
Box Jump Height: 24/20

PARTNER WOD 12
4 Rounds
50-Yard Kettlebell Farmers Carry (70/53)
10 Slamball Ground-Over-Shoulder (100/70)
15 Deadlifts (225/155)
20 Calorie Row
Buy-in/Buy-out: 21 Synchronized Air Squats

PARTNER WOD 13
16 Alternating Rounds
5 Power Cleans (135/95)
7 Push-ups
9 Air Squats
Buy-in/Buy-out: 150 Double-unders

PARTNER WOD 14
100 Double-unders
80 Wall Balls (24/20)
60 Power Snatches (95/65)
40 Over-the-Bar Burpees
50 Chest-to-Bar Pull-ups 60 Overhead Squats (95/65) 80 Wall Balls (24/20)
100 Double-unders

PARTNER WOD 15
63-45-27
Deadlifts (225/155)
Calorie Row
*75-Yard Slam Ball Bear Hug Carry After Every Round (100/70

PARTNER WOD 16
50 Alternating Dumbbell Snatches (55/35)
50 Calorie Bike

100 Wall Balls
100 Pull-ups

50 Calorie Bike
50 Alternating Dumbbell Snatches (55/35)

PARTNER WOD 17

1000 Meter Row
50 Deadlifts (185/130)
40 Toes-to-Bar

800 Meter Row
40 Deadlifts (225/155)
30 Toes-to-Bar

600 Meter Row
30 Deadlifts (275/190)
20 Toes-to-Bar

PARTNER WOD 18

70 Calorie Row
50 Thrusters (95/65)

60 Calorie Row
40 Thrusters (115/80)

50 Calorie Row
30 Thrusters (135/95)

40 Calorie Row
20 Thrusters (155/110)

PARTNER WOD 19

16 Deadlifts (275/190)
400 Meter Partner Run
80 Toes-to- Bar

14 Deadlifts (295/205)
400 Meter Partner Run
60 Burpee Box Jump Overs (24/20)

12 Deadlifts (315/220)
400 Meter Partner Run
40 Deficit Handstand Push-ups

PARTNER WOD 20
800 Meter Partner Run
60 Pull-ups
60 Deadlifts (185/130)

80 Calorie Bike
12 15' Rope Climbs
30 Power Cleans (185/130)

1600 Meter Row
100 Synchronized Air Squats
60 3' Burpee Broad Jumps

PARTNER WOD 21
6 Rounds
50-Yard Moderate Weight Sled Push
100 Double-unders
50 Wall Balls (20/14)

PARTNER WOD 22
20 Rounds
6 Power Cleans (135/95)
8 Chest-to-Bar Pull-ups
10 Calorie Row

PARTNER WOD 23
4 Rounds
400 Meter Run
20 Deadlifts (225/155)
25 Box Jumps (30/24)
30 GHD Sit-ups
35 Calorie Bike
40 Handstand Push-ups

PARTNER WOD 24
100 Power Cleans (135/95)
100 Burpees
100 Back Squats (135/95)
100 Kettlebell Swings (70/53)

PARTNER WOD 25
75 Snatches (75/55)
20 Box Jumps

65 Thrusters (95/65)
20 Box Jumps

55 Hang Cleans (135/95)
20 Box Jumps

45 Deadlifts (225/155)
20 Box Jumps
Box Jump Height: 24/20

PARTNER WOD 26
60 Power Snatches (115/80)
60 Calorie Row

50 Power Snatches (135/95)
50 Calorie Row

40 Power Snatches (155/110)
40 Calorie Row

PARTNER WOD 27
8 Rounds
10 Deadlifts (315/220)
20 Calorie Row
30 Calorie Bike

PARTNER WOD 28
4 Rounds
400 Meter Partner Run
10 Synchronized Clean + Jerks (185/130)
20 Synchronized Burpees
30-Yard Handstand Walk
40 Kettlebell Swings (70/53)

PARTNER WOD 29
3 Rounds
6 15' Rope Climbs
30-Yard Overhead Walking Lunges (Every 10 Yards 8 Synchronized Bar Facing Over-the-Bar Burpees)
10 Complexes of 1 Squat Snatch + 1 Hang Power Snatch
100 Dubs
Bar Weight: 135/95

PARTNER WOD 30
30 Deadlifts
30 Calorie Bike
20 Cleans
20 Burpee Box Jump Overs
10 Thrusters
20 Burpee Box Jump Overs
20 Cleans
30 Calorie Bike
30 Deadlifts
Bar Weight: 225/155
Box Height: 24/20

PARTNER WOD 31

Bike + Row: 30 + 35 Calories*
16 Complexes of 1 Squat Clean + 1 Front Squat (185/130)

Bike + Row: 25 + 30 Calories*
12 Complexes of 1 Squat Clean + 1 Front Squat (215/150)

Bike + Row: 20 + 25 Calories*
8 Complexes of 1 Squat Clean + 1 Front Squat Complex (245/170)
Both partners working at the same time, one partner bikes while the other rows. You may switch any time.

PARTNER WOD 32

21-15-9*
Thrusters (95/65)
Toes-to-Bar
Partner 1 completes the round of 21, then partner 2 completes the round of 21. Continue this same pattern for the rounds of 15 and 9.

PARTNER WOD 33

100 Wall Balls (20/14)
200 Double-unders

100 Calorie Row
200 Double-unders

100-Yard Handstand Walk
200 Double-unders

PARTNER WOD 34
4 Rounds
400 Meter Partner Run
16 Squat Cleans (185/130)

PARTNER WOD 35
1000 Meter Row

-straight into-

12 Alternating Rounds
5 Deadlifts (225/155)
10 Wall Balls (30/20)

-straight into-

800 Meter Row

-straight into-

10 Alternating Rounds
5 Goblet Squat (70/53)
10 Kettlebell Sumo Deadlift High Pull (70/53)

-straight into-

600 Meter Row

-straight into-

8 Alternating Rounds
5 Deadlifts (225/155)
5 Goblet Squat (70/53)

PARTNER WORKOUT 36
50-40-30-20-10
Calorie Bike
Deadlifts (185/130)
Non-working partner must hold a plank position. Switch every time one partner drops the bar or the plank position.

PARTNER WOD 37
9 Minute AMRAP
Minutes 1-4, AMRAP of
Complex:
3 Power Cleans
3 Shoulder-to-Overhead
3 Front Squats
Bar Weight: (135/95)
-Bar cannot be dropped once you begin the complex.
-Athlete may perform complex as many times as they'd like.
-Only 1 athlete working at a time.

Minutes 4-9, AMRAP of
Kettlebell Swings (70/53)

PARTNER WOD 38
30 Squat Cleans (135/95)
20 Over-the-Bar Burpees
100 Double-unders

24 Squat Cleans (185/130)
20 Over-the-Bar Burpees
100 Double-unders

18 Squat Cleans (225/155)
20 Over-the-Bar Burpees
100 Double-unders

12 Squat Cleans (275/180)
20 Over-the-Bar Burpees
100 Double-unders

PARTNER WOD 39
20 Squat Snatches
24 Synchronized Burpees

15 Squat Snatches
20 Synchronized Burpees

10 Squat Snatches
16 Synchronized Burpees

15 Squat Snatches
12 Synchronized Burpees

20 Squat Snatches
8 Synchronized Burpees
Bar Weight: 135/95

PARTNER WOD 40
1000 Meter Row*
50 Overhead Squats
50 GHD Sit-ups
8 15' Rope Climbs

800 Meter Row*
40 Overhead Squats
40 GHD Sit-ups
6 15' Rope Climbs

600 Meter Row*
30 Overhead Squats
30 GHD Sit-ups
4 15' Rope Climbs
Bar Weight: 115/80
*During each row, non-working partner much hold bar (115/80) in the overhead position.

PARTNER WOD 41
50 Thrusters
10 15' Rope Climbs

40 Thrusters
8 15' Rope Climbs

30 Thrusters
6 15' Rope Climbs

20 Thrusters
4 15' Rope Climbs
Bar Weight: (95/65)

PARTNER WOD 42
14 Minute AMRAP
10 Man Makers (40/30)
15 Box Jumps (24/20)
20 Overhead Squats (115/80)

PARTNER WOD 43
2 Rounds
50 Calorie Bike
40 Slamball Ground to Over-the-Shoulder
50 Dumbbell Shoulder-to-Overhead (50/35)*
40 Slamball Bear Hug Front Squats
Slamball Weight: 100/70
*Use two dumbbell for the shoulder-to-overhead.

PARTNER WOD 44
15 Minute AMRAP*
6 Thrusters (95/65)
6 Pull-ups
6 Burpees
*Alternating rounds

PARTNER WOD 45
60 Deadlifts
800 Meter Row

50 Power Cleans
700 Meter Row

40 Shoulder-to-Overhead
600 Meter Row

30 Deadlifts
500 Meter Row

20 Power Cleans
400 Meter Row

10 Shoulder-to-Overhead
300 Meter Row
Bar Weight: 135/95

PARTNER WOD 46
100 Meter Row
60 Back Squats
40 Box Jumps
20 GHD Sit-ups
10 Synchronized Over-the-Bar Burpees

800 Meter Row
50 Back Squats
30 Box Jumps
20 GHD Sit-ups
10 Synchronized Over-the-Bar Burpees

600 Meter Row
40 Back Squats
20 Box Jumps
10 Synchronized Over-the-Bar Burpees
Back Squats: 135/95
Box Jumps: 24/20

PARTNER WOD 47
30 Squat Snatches
40 Over-the-Bar Burpees
60 Pull-ups
40 Over-the-Bar Burpees
30 Squat Snatches
Bar Weight: 135/95

PARTNER WOD 48
10 Squat Cleans + Jerks
20 Chest-to-Bar Pull-ups
30 Toes-to- Bar
40 Bike Calories
30 Toes-to- Bar
20 Chest-to-Bar Pull-ups
10 Squat Cleans + Jerks
Bar Weight: 235/165

PARTNER WOD 49
3 Rounds
400 Meter Med Ball Run (20/14)*
50 Dumbbell Shoulder-to-Overhead (50/35)*
40 GHD Sit-ups
*1 med ball per team.
*2 Dumbbells for the shoulder-to-overhead.

PARTNER WOD 50
10 Dumbbell Squat Snatches, Alternating Hands (50/30)
10 Chest-to-Bar Pull-ups
*Switch working partner every minute on the minute.

PARTNER WOD 51
200 Double-unders
21 Squat Snatches

100 Double-unders
15 Squat Snatches

50 Double-unders
9 Squat Snatches
Bar Weight: 135/95

PARTNER WOD 52
2 Clean + Jerks (135/95)
2 Synchronized Burpees
2 Pull-Ups
4 Clean + Jerks
4 Synchronized Burpees
4 Pull-Ups
-Continue this pattern, adding 2 reps to each rep every round.
-Finish at the round of 16.

PARTNER WOD 53
20 Synchronized Kettlebell Deadlifts (70/53)*
30 Hand-Release Push-ups
40 Dumbbell Snatches, Alternating Hands (50/35)
50 Toes-to-Bar
60 Synchronized Air Squats
50 Toes-to-Bar
40 Dumbbell Snatches, Alternating Hands (50/35)
30 Hand-Release Push-ups
20 Synchronized Kettlebell Deadlifts (70/53)*
*One kettlebell in each hand.

PARTNER WOD 54

80 Calorie Row
60 Synchronized Burpees

70 Calorie Row
50 Synchronized Burpees

60 Calorie Row
40 Synchronized Burpees

50 Calorie Row
30 Synchronized Burpees

40 Calorie Row
20 Synchronized Burpees

30 Calorie Row
10 Synchronized Burpees

PARTNER WOD 55

24 Deadlifts (185/130)
48 Dumbbell Shoulder-to-Overhead*

24 Deadlifts (185/130)
48 Hand-release Push-ups*

24 Deadlifts
48 Pull-ups*

Deadlift: 185/130
Dumbbell: 50/35 (use two dumbbells)
*Non-working partner must hold deadlift bar at the top of the deadlift position. Switch every time the bar is dropped.

PARTNER WOD 56
80 Wall Balls (24/20)
70 Kettlebell Sumo Deadlift High Pulls (70/53)
60 Calorie Row
50 Overhead Squats (95/65)
40 Pull-ups
30 Handstand Push-ups
20 Synchronized Burpees
10 Man-Makers (30/20)

CHAPTER 9
CHIPPERS

Chippers are one-round workouts that generally include many different movements performed at high reps. For the most part, chippers are aerobically intensive workouts—often considered to be the most mentally challenging because they tend to *chip away* at you, slowly taxing your psyche and your body. Of course, it can also be said that you're the one *chipping away* at the workout—a matter of perspective I guess! Chippers are great for learning to pace, developing mental fortitude, an aerobic base, muscular endurance, burning fat, and for testing your technique under fatigue. Consider Chipper Workout 2 for example, a series for high rep barbell movements sandwiched by gymnastics exercises:

60 Power Cleans
50 Burpees
40 Shoulder-to-Overhead
30 Toes-to-Bar
20 Power Snatches
10 Ring Muscle-ups
Bar Weight: 95/65

Tips for Tackling a Chipper
1. Scale accordingly. Scaling a chipper workout can be somewhat deceiving since most are already programmed with relatively light weight. However, there's a reason for this. Chipper Workout 2, for example, begins with power cleans at 95/65—for most people, that's not a very heavy weight. The catch is that you'll have to perform 60 reps! Consider how much your form and speed will decline once you begin to fatigue—and that's only the first part of the workout. If you don't have much experience with chipper workouts, it pays to be conservative. As a general rule, aim to scale your bar weight to 50%

or less of your one-rep max.

2. Manage your rest periods. Managing your rest periods is a crucial part of any workout, but it's especially true in a chipper workout. Because of the high-rep scheme of a chipper workout, you'll likely take more breaks than you would in any other type of workout. As such, resting just five seconds more than necessary on every break can add up to minutes once the workout is complete.

3. Have a plan. If you're going to take your time coming up with a plan of attack for any workout, it's going to be a chipper! Focus on managing your heart rate. This isn't the type of WOD that should spike your heart rate two minutes into the workout. If that happens, you're in for a world of suffering. Instead, stay the conservative path with small sets early on in the workout. If half way through the WOD you feel like you can turn it up a notch and move on to bigger sets, go for it. If you burn out, at least you'll already be half way done with the workout.

CHIPPER WOD 1

60 Double-unders
50 Air Squats
40 Power Snatches (75/55)
30 Burpees
20 Chest-to-Bar Pull-ups
10 15' Rope Climbs

CHIPPER WOD 2

60 Power Cleans
50 Burpees
40 Shoulder-to-Overhead
30 Toes-to-Bar
20 Power Snatches
10 Ring Muscle-ups
Bar Weight: 95/65

CHIPPER WOD 3

50 Wall Balls (20/14)
50 Calorie Row
40 Pull-ups
40 Deadlifts (225/155)
30 Goblet Squats (70/53)
30 Alternating Dumbbell Snatches (55/40)
20 Over-the-Bar Burpees
20 Alternating Pistols

CHIPPER WOD 4

1.5 Mile Run
50 Thrusters (95/65)
50 Toes-to-Bar
50 Calorie Row
50 Ring Dips

CHIPPER WOD 5
800 Meter Med Ball Run (20/14)
60 Power Cleans (115/80)
50 Handstand Push-ups
40 Kettlebell Swings (70/53)
30 Chest-to-Bar Pull-ups
20 Box Jumps (24/20)
10 3' Burpee Broad Jumps

CHIPPER WOD 6
10 Bar Muscle-Ups
20 Wall Balls (30/20)
30 Calorie Bike
40 Air Squats
50 Calorie Row
40 Air Squats
30 Calorie Bike
20 Wall Balls (30/20)
10 Bar Muscle-Ups

CHIPPER WOD 7
60 Overhead Squats
50 3' Burpee Broad Jumps
40 Clean + Jerks
30 Toes-to-Bar
20 Ring Dips
Bar Weight: 95/65

CHIPPER WOD 8
50 Front Squat
40 Burpees
30 Pull-ups
20 Push Presses
10 15' Rope Climbs
20 Push Presses
30 Pull-ups
40 Burpees
50 Front Squat
Bar Weight: 95/65

CHIPPER WOD 9
50 Kettlebell Swings (70/53)
50 Toes-to-Bar
50 Wall Balls (20/14)
50 Burpee Box Jump Overs (24/20)
50 Calorie Row
50 Double-unders
50 Handstand Push-ups

CHIPPER WOD 10
50 Alternating In-place Back Rack Lunges
40 Push Jerks
30 Toes-to-Bar
20 Squat Cleans
10 Ring Muscle-ups
Bar Weight: 135/95

CHIPPER WOD 11
20 Power Cleans (135/95)
20 Box Jumps (24/20)
20 Kettlebell Swings (70/53)
20 Bar Facing Over-the-Bar Burpees
100 Double-unders
20 Bar Facing Over-the-Bar Burpees
20 Kettlebell Swings (70/53)
20 Box Jumps (24/20)
20 Power Cleans (135/95)

CHIPPER WOD 12
40 Shoulder-to- Overhead
35 Russian Kettlebell Swings
30 Calorie Row
25 Power Snatches
20 Muscle-Ups
25 Power Snatches
30 Calorie Row
35 Russian Kettlebell Swings
40 Shoulder-to-Overhead
Bar Weight: 95/65
Kettlebell Weight: 70/53

CHIPPER WOD 13
40 Wall Balls (20/14)
30 Toes-to-Bar
20 Deadlifts (225/155)
10 Burpee Box Jump Overs (30/24)
20 Deadlifts (225/155)
30 Toes-to-Bar
40 Wall Balls (20/14)

CHIPPER WOD 14
100 Double-unders
40 Shoulder-to-Overhead
40 Box Jump Overs (24/20)
40 Overhead Squats
40 Toes-to- Bar
40 Power Cleans
100 Double-unders
Bar Weight: 115/80

CHIPPER WOD 15
10 Overhead Squats
20 Power Cleans
30 GHD Sit-ups
40 Russian Kettlebell Swings (70/53)
50 Double-unders
40 Russian Kettlebell Swings (70/53)
30 GHD Sit-ups
20 Power Cleans
10 Overhead Squats
Bar Weight: 115/80

CHIPPER WOD 16
24 Clean + Jerks
20 Calorie Row
16 Squat Snatches
14 Over-the-Bar Burpees
10 Ring Muscle-ups
14 Over-the-Bar Burpees
16 Squat Snatches
20 Calorie Row
24 Clean + Jerks
Bar Weight: 115/80

CHIPPER WOD 17
20 Deadlifts (185/130)
25 Box Jump Overs
30 Toes-to-Bar
35 Calorie Row
40 Alternating Hang Dumbbell Snatches (40/25)
45 Double-unders
50 Air Squats
45 Double-unders
40 Alternating Hang Dumbbell Snatches (40/25)
35 Calorie Row
30 Toes-to-Bar
25 Box Jump Overs
20 Deadlifts (185/130)

CHIPPER WOD 18
1 Mile Assault Bike
80 Air Squats
60 Power Snatches (75/55)
40 Burpee Box Jump Overs (24/20)
20 Toes-to-Bar
1 Mile Assault Bike

CHIPPER WOD 19
60 Wall Balls (20/14)
50 Calorie Row
40 Toes-to-Bar
30 GHD Sit-ups
20 Box Jumps (24/20)
10 Ring Muscle-ups
100 Double-unders

CHIPPER WOD 20
10 Squat Cleans (225/155)
20 Handstand Push-ups
30 Calorie Row
40 Chest-to-Bar Pull-ups
50 GHD Sit-ups
40 Chest-to-Bar Pull-ups
30 Calorie Row
20 Handstand Push-ups
10 Squat Cleans (225/155)

CHIPPER WOD 21
2000 Meter Row
50 Front Squats
50 Push-ups
50 Shoulder-to-Overhead
50 Ring Dips
50 Shoulder-to-Overhead
50 Push-ups
50 Front Squats
2000 Meter Row
Bar Weight: 95/65

CHIPPER WOD 22
35 Calorie Row
30 Burpees
25 Pull-ups
20 Handstand Push-ups
15 Box Jumps (30/24)
20 Handstand Push-ups
25 Pull-ups
30 Burpees
35 Calorie Row

CHIPPER WOD 23
10 Burpee Box Jump Overs (30/24)
20 Power Cleans
30 Calorie Row
40 Deadlifts
50 Russian Kettlebell Swings (70/53)
60 Air Squat
70 Double-unders
Bar Weight: 135/95

CHIPPER WOD 24
40 Handstand Push-ups
40 Calorie Row
40 Chest-to-Bar Pull-ups
40 Shoulder-to-Overhead (135/95)

CHIPPER WOD 25
50 Wall Balls (20/14)
40 Chest-to-Bar Pull-ups
30 Calorie Row
20 Alternating Front Rack Dumbbell Lunges (50/35)
100 Double-unders

CHIPPER WOD 26
50 Deadlifts (205/145)
50 Toes-to-Bar
50 Alternating Dumbbell Snatches (50/35)
50 Push-ups
50 Russian Kettlebell Swings (70/53)

CHAPTERS 10A/10B
RUNNING

The workouts in this chapter have one thing in common, they all incorporate running. Most functional fitness athletes fall into one of two categories: they either hate running or they love it. And, if they love running, it's usually because they've had some other relationship to it such as training for marathons or competing in track and field. There's something to be said about that. In short, the more you run, the more you'll like it—hopefully!

Most of the WODs in this chapter will have you run between 100 meters and 1 mile at any given time. I've divided this chapter into two parts: traditional WODs (couplets, triplets, AMRAPs, etc.) with some running element and long interval running WODs. The long interval running WODs are probably the most unique WODs you'll see in this book. In general, these WODs usually take at least 40 minutes to complete. As such, they shouldn't be programmed more than once every one or two weeks. I've done them all and can honestly tell you they're a ton of fun—and extremely brutal!

Note: Several of the long interval running WODs (Long Interval Running WOD 1, for example) call for you to increase the weight on a specific movement each interval. Weight changes should be made during the rest period of your interval.

RUNNING WOD 1
3 Rounds
400 Meter Run
15 Squat Cleans (185/130)
15 Burpee Box Jump Overs (24/20)

RUNNING WOD 2
400 Meter Run
50 Russian Kettlebell Swings

-rest 1 minute-

400 Meter Run
40 Russian Kettlebell Swings

-rest 1 minute-

400 Meter Run
30 Russian Kettlebell Swings
Kettlebell Weight: 70/53

RUNNING WOD 3
12 Minute AMRAP
5 Squat Snatches (135/95)
10 Chest-to-Bar Pull-ups
400 Meter Run

RUNNING WOD 4
3 Rounds
400 Meter Run
25-Yard Moderate Weight Sled Push
20-Yard Overhead Walking Lunges (95/65)
15 Russian Kettlebell Swings (70/53)

RUNNING WOD 5

30 Kettlebell Swings
40 Wall Balls
400 Meter Run with Med Ball

20 Kettlebell Swings
30 Wall Balls
400 Meter Run with Med Ball

10 Kettlebell Swings
20 Wall Balls
400 Meter Run with Med Ball
Kettlebell Weight: 70/53
Med Ball Weight: 20/14

RUNNING WOD 6

15 Minute AMRAP
200 Meter Run
12 Deadlifts (225/155)
8 Burpee Box Jump Overs (24/20)
6 Handstand Push-ups

RUNNING WOD 7

21-15-9
Power Snatches (95/65)
Pull-ups
Wall Balls (20/14)
GHD Sit-ups
*400 Meter Run Before Every Round

RUNNING WOD 8
1 Mile Run
60 Wall Balls (20/14)
45 Overhead Squats (95/65)
30 Burpee Box Jump Overs (24/20)

RUNNING WOD 9
3 Rounds
15 Shoulder-to-Overhead
400 Meter run
12 Overhead Squats
9 Chest-to-Bar Pull-ups
30 Double-unders
Bar Weight: 115/80

RUNNING WOD 10
For Time
1,000 Meter Row
400 Meter Run
500 Meter Row
400 Meter Run

RUNNING WOD 11
3 Rounds
400 Meter Run
14 Alternating Dumbbell Snatches
2 Man Makers
14 Dumbbell Push Presses
2 Man Makers
14 Dumbbell Front Rack Squats
2 Man Makers
Dumbbell Weight: 40/30
*One dumbbell in each arm.

RUNNING WOD 12
1 Mile Run
50 Power Cleans (135/95)
40 Pull-ups
30 Kettlebell Swings (53/35)
20 3' Burpee Broad Jumps
10 Man-makers (40/30)

RUNNING WOD 13
3 Rounds
25-Yard Moderate Weight Sled Push
30 Double-unders
400 Meter Run
12 Alternating Dumbbell Squat Snatches (50/35)
12 Burpees
Buy-out: 15 Muscle-ups or 30 Chest-to-Bar Pull-ups

RUNNING WOD 14
21-15-9
Power Cleans
Calorie Bike
Shoulder-to-Overhead
GHD Sit-ups
*400 Meter Run Before Every Round
Bar Weight: 135/95

RUNNING WOD 15
4 Rounds
400 Meter Run
25 GHD Sit-ups

RUNNING WOD 16
800 Meter Run
40 Back Squats
30 Box Jumps (24/20)
20 Power Cleans
10 15' Rope Climbs
800 Meter Run
Barbell Weight: 135/95

RUNNING WOD 17
6 Rounds
100 Meter Sprint
10 3' Burpee Broad Jumps
12 Thrusters (95/65)

RUNNING WOD 18
12 Minute AMRAP
5 Squat Snatches (135/95)
10 Chest-to-Bar Pull-ups
400 Meter Run

RUNNING WOD 19
3 Rounds
400 Meter Run
20 Power Cleans (135/95)
15 Handstand Push-ups

CHAPTER 11B
LONG INTERVAL RUNNING WODS

LONG INTERVAL RUNNING WOD 1
400 Meter Run
15 Squat Cleans (135/95)
30 Double-unders
15 Handstand Push-ups
25-Yard Double Kettlebell Overhead Lunges (40/30)

-rest 2 minutes-

400 Meter Run
12 Squat Cleans (185/130)
30 Double-unders
15 Handstand Push-ups
25-Yard Double Kettlebell Overhead Lunges (40/30)

-rest 2 minutes-

400 Meter Run
9 Squat Cleans (225/155)
30 Double-unders
15 Handstand Push-ups
25-Yard Double Kettlebell Overhead Lunges (40/30)

LONG INTERVAL RUNNING WOD 2

600 Meter Run
21 Power Cleans
21 Wall Balls
21 Pull-Ups

-rest 1.5 minutes-

400 Meter Run
15 Power Cleans
15 Wall Balls
15 Pull-Ups

-rest 1 minute-

200 Meter Run
9 Power Cleans
9 Wall Balls
9 Pull-Ups
Bar Weight: 135/95
Wall Balls: 20/14

LONG INTERVAL RUNNING WOD 3

400 Meter Run
30 Wall Balls
30 Toes-to-Bar
30 Power Cleans
30 GHD Sit-ups

-rest 2 minutes-

500 Meter Row
20 Wall Balls
20 Toes-to-Bar
20 Power Cleans
20 GHD Sit-ups

-rest 2 minutes-

400 Meter Run
10 Wall Balls
10 Toes-to-Bar
10 Power Cleans
10 GHD Sit-ups
Bar Weight: 115/80
Wall Balls: 20/14

LONG INTERVAL RUNNING WOD 4

400 Meter Run
30 Deadlifts (225/155)
40 Wall Balls (20/14)
20 Toes-to-Bar
20 Goblet Squats (70/53)

-rest 2 minutes-

400 Meter Run
20 Deadlifts (225/155)
30 Wall Balls (20/14)
20 Toes-to-Bar
20 Goblet Squats (70/53)

-rest 1.5 minutes-

400 Meter Run
10 Deadlifts (225/155)
20 Wall Balls (20/14)
20 Toes-to-Bar
20 Goblet Squats (70/53)

LONG INTERVAL RUNNING WOD 5
10 Thrusters (135/95)
15 Over-the-Bar Burpees
20 Deadlifts (135/95)
25 Russian Kettlebell Swings (70/53)
400 Meter Run

-rest 1.5 minutes-

10 Thrusters (165/115)
15 Over-the-Bar Burpees
20 Deadlifts
25 Russian Kettlebell Swings
400 Meter Run

-rest 1.5 minutes-

10 Thrusters (195/135)
15 Over-the-Bar Burpees
20 Deadlifts
25 Russian Kettlebell Swings
400 Meter Run

LONG INTERVAL RUNNING WOD 6
400 Meter Run
15 Squat Cleans (135/95)
30 Double-unders
15 Handstand Push-ups
24 In-place Kettlebell Lunges (40/30)*

-rest 2 minutes-

400 Meter Run
13 Squat Cleans (185/130)
30 Double-unders
15 Handstand Push-ups

24 In-place Kettlebell Lunges (40/30)*

-rest 2 minutes-

400 Meter Run
11 Squat Cleans (225/155)
30 Double-unders
15 Handstand Push-ups
24 In-place Kettlebell Lunges (40/30)*
*Use two kettlebells in the front rack position.

LONG INTERVAL RUNNING WOD 7
600 Meter Run
5 Complexes of 1 Power Clean, 1 Hang Squat Clean, 1 Front Squat, 1 Shoulder-to-Overhead (135/95)
20 Box Jump Overs
20 Kettlebell Swings

-rest 2 minutes-

400 Meter Run
5 Complexes of 1 Power Clean, 1 Hang Squat Clean, 1 Front Squat, 1 Shoulder-to-Overhead (165/115)
16 Box Jump Overs
16 Kettlebell Swings

-rest 1.5 minutes-

600 Meter Run
5 Complexes of 1 Power Clean, 1 Hang Squat Clean, 1 Front Squat, 1 Shoulder-to-Overhead (185/130)
12 Box Jump Overs
12 Kettlebell Swings

-rest 1 minute-

400 Meter Run

5 Complexes of 1 Power Clean, 1 Hang Squat Clean, 1 Front Squat, 1 Shoulder-to-Overhead (205/145)
8 Box Jump Overs
8 Kettlebell Swings
Box Jump Height: 24/20
Kettebell Weight: 70/53

LONG INTERVAL RUNNING WOD 8
400 Meter Run
30 Thrusters
500 Meter Row
21 Chest-to-Bar Pull-ups
21 Power Snatches
21 Box Jumps

-rest 2 minutes-

400 Meter Run
20 Thrusters
500 Meter Row
15 Chest-to-Bar Pull-ups
15 Power Snatches
15 Box Jumps

-rest 2 minutes-

400 Meter Run
10 Thrusters
500 Meter Row
9 Chest-to-Bar Pull-ups
9 Power Snatches
9 Box Jumps
Bar Weight: 95/65
Box Height: 24/20

LONG INTERVAL RUNNING WOD 9

400 Meter Run
21 Power Cleans
21 Pull-ups
21 Toes-to-Bar
21 Kettlebell Swings
21 Over-the-Bar Burpees

-rest 2 minutes-

400 Meter Run
21 Power Snatches
15 Pull-ups
15 Toes-to-Bar
15 Kettlebell Swings
15 Over-the-Bar Burpees

-rest 1.5 minutes-

400 Meter Run
21 Thrusters
9 Pull-ups
9 Toes-to-Bar
9 Kettlebell Swings
9 Over-the-Bar Burpees

-rest 1 minute-

400 Meter Run
21 Overhead Squats
6 Pull-ups
6 Toes-to-Bar
6 Kettlebell Swings
6 Over-the-Bar Burpees
Bar Weight: 135/95
Kettlebell Weight: 75/53

LONG INTERVAL RUNNING WOD 10

800 Meter Run
20 Power Cleans (135/95)
5 Man Makers
10 Burpee Box Jump Overs
15 Chest-to-Bar Pull-ups
20 Toes-to-Bar

-rest 1.5 minutes-

600 Meter Run
15 Power Cleans (155/110)
5 Man Makers
10 Burpee Box Jump Overs
15 Chest-to-Bar Pull-ups
20 Toes-to-Bar

-rest 1.5 minutes-

400 Meter Run
10 Power Cleans (175/125)
5 Man Makers
10 Burpee Box Jump Overs
15 Chest-to-Bar Pull-ups
20 Toes-to-Bar
Man Maker Dumbbell Weight: 30/20
Box Jump Height: 24/20

LONG INTERVAL RUNNING WOD 11
30 Deadlifts
20 Power Snatches
400 Meter Run
30 GHD Sit-ups
20 Shoulder-to-Overhead

-rest 2 minutes-

25 Deadlifts
15 Power Snatches
400 Meter Run
25 GHD Sit-ups
15 Shoulder-to-Overhead

-rest 1.5 minutes-

20 Deadlifts
10 Power Snatches
400 Meter Run
20 GHD Sit-ups
10 Shoulder-to-Overhead
Bar Weight: 135/95

LONG INTERVAL RUNNING WOD 12

800 Meter Run
10 Clean + Jerks (185/130)
15 Over-the-Bar Burpees
20 Handstand Push-ups

-rest 2 minutes-

600 Meter Run
8 Clean + Jerks (205/145)
12 Over-the-Bar Burpees
16 Handstand Push-ups

-rest 1.5 minutes-

400 Meter Run
6 Clean + Jerks (225/155)
9 Over-the-Bar Burpees
12 Handstand Push-ups

"Adapt what is useful, reject what is useless, and add what is specifically your own."
-Bruce Lee

TRAINING DAY